DUTY AND HEALING

foundations of a jewish bioethic

Reflective Bioethics

Series Editors:
Hilde Lindemann Nelson and James Lindemann Nelson

The Patient in the Family
Hilde Lindemann Nelson and James Lindemann Nelson

Do We Still Need Doctors?
John D. Lantos, M.D.

Stories and Their Limits: Narrative Approaches to Bioethics
Hilde Lindemann Nelson

Physician Assisted Suicide: Expanding the Debate
Rosamond Rhodes, Margaret P. Battin, Anita Silvers, eds.

A Philosophical Disease
Carl Elliott

The Fiction of Bioethics:
Cases as Literary Texts
Tod Chambers

Meaning and Medicine:
A Reader in the Philosophy of Health Care
James Lindemann Nelson and Hilde Lindemann Nelson, eds.

DUTY AND HEALING

foundations of a jewish bioethic

Benjamin Freedman

with an Introduction by
Charles Weijer

ROUTLEDGE

New York London

Published in 1999 by
Routledge
29 West 35th Street
New York, NY 10001

Published in Great Britain by
Routledge
11 New Fetter Lane
London EC4P 4EE

Library of Congress Cataloging-in-Publication Data

Freedman, Benjamin
    Duty and healing: foundations of a Jewish bioethic / Benjamin Freedman; Charles Weijer, ed.
      p. cm. — (Reflective bioethics)
    Includes bibliographical references and index.
    ISBN 0-415-92179-1. — ISBN 0-415-92180-5 (pbk.)
    1. Bioethics — Religious aspects — Judaism. 2. Bioethics. 3. Medical laws and legislation
(Jewish Law) 4. Ethics, Jewish. I. Weijer, Charles. II. Title. III. Series.
BM538.H43F74 1999
296.3'642—dc21   98-40642
                                                                                                           CIP

CONTENTS

SECTION 3

COMPETENCY

Jewish Sources and the General Theory of Competency

SECTION 4

RISK

Principles of Judgment in Health Care Decisions

AFTERWORD

Next Steps in Healing and Duty

Editor's Introduction

R El'azar ben Shamu'a says, Let the honor of your student be as dear to you as your own, and the honor of your fellow as the honor of your teacher, and the honor of your teacher as the awe of Heaven.

—Pirkei Avot, Chapter 4, Mishna 15

Benjamin Freedman, one of the foremost thinkers in bioethics, died from complications of palliative surgery for stomach cancer on March 20, 1997, 12 Adar II, at forty-six years of age. A productive and dedicated scholar to the end, he asked four of his closest colleagues, Françoise Baylis, Kathleen Cranley Glass, Robert J. Levine, and myself, to ensure that his unfinished work was completed and that unpublished manuscripts were brought to press. As a result of discussions with this group and his widow (and literary executor), Barbara Freedman, the task of bringing this book, *Duty and Healing: Foundations of a Jewish Bioethic,* Benjy's last major work and the project most dear to him, to publication fell to me. A straw poll of friends and colleagues who know much more about books than I do revealed a universal antipathy to lengthy introductions from editors. I will, therefore, be brief and contain my comments to the genesis of this book, the man who wrote it, and the debts of gratitude I incurred while editing it.

The Book

As both an Orthodox Jew and a philosopher, Benjy described feeling for many years a rift between his spiritual and professional lives. This gap began to be bridged in 1987 when he took up the positions of clinical bioethicist at the Sir Mortimer B. Davis Jewish General Hospital and Professor of Medicine and Philosophy in the Biomedical Ethics Unit at McGill University. Working in a hospital in which 40% of the patient population were religious Jews meant that clinical consultations often called upon his knowledge of both bioethics and Jewish law. The final impetus for Benjy to begin this book, a synthesis of bioethics and Jewish law is, in retrospect, bitterly ironic:

> A few years into this process, a terrifying and wonderful event occurred. A chest X ray indicated a possible malignancy. For a bit over a day, I lived with the knowledge that, in the words of my doctor, "This is probably nothing, but it could be very, very bad." Such a conversation concentrates the mind wonderfully. Thinking through a long night about what could come next, I found, to my surprise, that my chief regret was that I had never put down in writing my thoughts and work on Judaism and bioethics. That sense stayed with me after learning that the whole thing had been a false alarm. Subsequently, I worked when I could on Jewish sources, and devoted myself to writing a book on this throughout my sabbatical year.
>
> My original and continuing motivation, then, was to complete this work and to make it as widely available, for as long a time, as possible. Fulfilling these tasks, to my mind, is like fulfilling a vow—in this case, both a personal and a religious obligation. (http://www.mcgill.ca/ctrg/bfreed/whyweb.html)

On one level, *Duty and Healing* is an essay on the application of a regime of duties to the moral issues that arise in contemporary health care; on another level, however, the book is itself an expression of Benjy's own sense of duty and the healing that finally joined his faith and his profession.

Benjy completed *Duty and Healing* in 1996. From the start, his intention was to make the book available on the Internet, rather than through a publisher. Despite the efforts of a number of colleagues, myself included, to convince him otherwise, Benjy finally elected to "publish" the book on the Internet for several reasons. The Internet allowed him to make the book available immediately to users of libraries around the world and millions of people with home computers and modems. No compromises would have to be made with a publisher; the book could be whatever length he wished, and technical material could be relegated to endnotes and appendices, rather than eliminated. Finally, the book could be added to and, if necessary, altered as his own work evolved. The Internet version of the book received excellent reviews in a variety of journals, including the prestigious *Journal of the American Medical Association,* and many colleagues quietly admired his decision to publish it in the way he did.

Shortly after Benjy's death, the opportunity to publish *Duty and Healing* in hard copy came up unexpectedly. At the Annual Bioethics Summer Retreat in 1997, I had dinner with John Lantos and Jim and Hilde Nelson. John suggested that Benjy's book would make a fine addition to the Reflections in Bioethics series that Jim and Hilde edit for Routledge, and they enthusiastically agreed. When I approached Barbara Freedman about the idea, I discovered that she and her family were anxious to see the book in print. While the Internet made the book available to many, they were worried that few would actually print out and read the entire five-hundred-page manuscript. Also, while most in academia have access to the Internet, only a minority of the population at large does—perhaps 10% at the time of writing. Finally, it was unlikely that the book would be used to educate the next generation of scholars unless available in printed form. In short, the family felt that Benjy's legacy would be better served by a printed book than one solely available in cyberspace.

The book, in its present form, has been shortened by about 20% in length from the Internet version. Explanatory endnotes, some in excess of two pages in length in the original, were cut to one or two sentences. Endnotes from which material has been removed are indicated with an asterisk (*). Appendices, which contain discussions of interest to a specialist audience, were taken out of this volume. To ensure that all of these materials remain available to the interested reader, however, they have been placed on a website (http://www.mcgill.ca/ctrg/bfreed), and this site may be accessed through the website of Routledge. On the website, the endnotes are arranged in parallel with the main divisions of the book, and their numbering corresponds to that found in the book. The appendices are also arranged by section and are as follows:

- Section 1: Family
  - Appendix 1: Reward and Reciprocity, Parent and Child: Commentary on *Ty Pei'a* 1.1
- Section 2: Consent
  - Appendix 1: Coercion to Undergo Treatment
  - Appendix 2: A Rabbinic Example of Required Consent
  - Appendix 3: Two Objections to the Caretaker Model Rebutted
  - Appendix 4: A Rabbinic Discussion of Barriers to Consent
- Section 4: Risk
  - Appendix 1: Participation in Clinical Research: Convergence of Jewish and Contemporary Perspectives
  - Appendix 2: Risk-Benefit Rationality and *Halakhic* Discontinuities: *Terefa* and *Goses*

Only a few minor changes were made to the main text of the book: Some punctuation was added or changed, and a number of sentences were reworded for clarity. Finally, a list of sources of Jewish law, a glossary of terms, and an index were added to the book to assist the reader.

The Author

The passing of Benjamin Freedman was marked in many ways by his colleagues in bioethics. Laurie Zoloth-Dorfman and Sue Rubin organized a session in his honor at the Society for Health and Human Values meeting in Baltimore, Gerry Batist gathered seven colleagues from across North America to present papers in honor of Benjy at the Sir Mortimer B. Davis Jewish General Hospital in Montreal (these papers are currently being collected for publication), and another tribute was made by Laurie Zoloth-Dorfman in the presentation and discussion of this book at the First International Conference of Jewish Bioethics. Benjy was remembered in a number of in memoriam pieces, each presenting its own perspective on his life and his work.[1]

My own professional relationship and friendship with Benjy began in the spring of 1991. Already a physician, I had just completed the first year of a bachelor's degree in philosophy at McGill University. Unable to practice medicine in Quebec, I was, at the time, searching rather urgently for a job. I met Benjy to interview for the position of research assistant funded by a grant he and colleagues Abe Fuks and Stan Shapiro had just received to investigate ethical issues in cancer clinical trials (the beginning of what is now the Clinical Trials Research Group). At the start of the interview he asked me how my last name was pronounced. "*VEY-er*" I replied. "I see," he said, "as in *oy veyz mir*"—a Yiddish expression of exasperation. Benjy's observations about people were almost always acute; in this case, it bordered on the prophetic.

For the remainder of the interview we retired to a kosher Moroccan restaurant run by a friend (and Cabalistic scholar). A novice to North African cuisine, I ordered *mergez,* a very spicy sausage dish, despite the cautions offered by Benjy and the owner. Our conversation over lunch was engaging, to say the least. After a while I forgot that I was being interviewed, and we drifted from one topic to the next: from the practice of medicine to my experiences working among first-nations peoples, from theories of mental illness to poetry. As our lunch, and the interview, drew to a close he offered me the job. I eagerly accepted. Some time later, I asked Benjy why he had hired me, and he insisted that he and Abe had agreed that I would be hired only if I ordered the *mergez*—a sure sign of intellectual adventurousness, he claimed. I remain fond of those spicy sausages to this day.

I feel privileged to have worked with Benjy for six years; in his twenty-two-year career as a bioethicist, he trained only two doctoral students, Françoise Baylis and myself. Benjy mentored his graduate students with the same paternal skill that he applied to his own children. At first, I retrieved and photocopied articles for the research group; later, I participated in developing and writing up projects;

finally, I ventured in my own direction in research. Taking my first steps into academia, I knew he was always watching, always close enough to prevent an embarrassing fall. Without question, he was a tough critic and demanding supervisor. My first attempt at writing was returned with a sticky note that read simply, "Truly bad." As hard to swallow as some comments were, he was very accurate in his criticism, and responding to it over the years made my work better. I learned that rigorous self-criticism is the essence of being a true scholar. Knowing that Benjy would not mince words, praise for my work from him meant more than praise from anyone else. I remember well the day that a paper of mine was returned with the single comment, "Terrific"—it was a graduation of sorts for me.

Indeed, Benjy's clarity of thought and academic rigor characterize his many seminal contributions to the field of bioethics. Early in his career, Benjy observed that the task of bioethics was "the exposure of muddled and wrong-headed concepts, to clear the way for a healthy growth of ideas."[2] In the six books and monographs and one hundred twenty-two articles that comprise his opus, he not only cleared the way, but also filled the gap with profoundly influential ideas. Reflecting on his work, the most remarkable aspect of it, to me at least, is the consistency of quality and originality. If truth be told, most of us in academia find ourselves reworking, at one time or another, the same idea in several different papers, and some papers are not among our best work. Not so with Benjy. Each of his books and papers was a true contribution to the literature; his work was all wheat and no chaff—a remarkable feat for such a productive scholar.

Benjy's early work explored the philosophical foundations of decision making by, or on behalf of, patients. Physicians have a duty to acknowledge valid consent from patients and, he argued, this implies a duty to respect a patient's wish not to be informed of the risks of a medical procedure—so-called ignorant consent.[3] When a patient is incapable of speaking for herself, a variety of approaches as to how a decision ought to be made on her behalf have been proposed. Benjy argued convincingly against the prevalent hypothetical test, deciding as the patient herself would have (how, after all, could one know?), and in favor of a best-interests approach.[4] Perhaps most difficult are those cases at the margin, when a patient is neither clearly capable nor clearly incapable of deciding for herself. Benjy proposed a novel standard of "recognizable reasons" by which a person is judged competent if able to supply premises that argue for a practical conclusion.[2-4] All of these issues are further explored in the context of Jewish law in Sections 1–3 of this book.

Benjy is perhaps best known for his work in the ethics of human experimentation. His concept of clinical equipoise is widely regarded as the moral foundation of the randomized controlled trial, crucial medical experiments in which patients are assigned by chance to an experimental treatment or a control treatment.[5] According to the concept, a trial may be initiated ethically only if there exists an honest, professional disagreement in the community of expert clinicians as to the preferred treatment. The purpose of the trial is to resolve this disagreement—in other words, to change clinical practice. The implications of clinical equipoise are far-reaching. Freedman was the first to recognize that ethical issues in clinical research extend to include aspects of the design of clinical trials.[6] For example, in the choice of a control treatment, clinical equipoise argues for the use of standard treatment, when such treatment exists, rather than a placebo, in part because the comparison of experimental and standard treatment is the most relevant to clinicians and patients (and, thus, more likely to influence the practice of physicians).[7]

Other work in research ethics clarifies the ethical analysis of the risks and benefits associated with study participation. Benjy recognized that not all interventions in research are performed with the same intention: Some are done with therapeutic intent, others serve only the scientific issue at hand. He and colleagues argued that therapeutic interventions must pass the test of clinical equipoise (a risk-benefit calculus).[8] Nontherapeutic interventions ("dedicated research interventions") must be weighed separately: The risks associated with them must be minimized, and risk must be proportionate to potential gains in knowledge from the study (a risk-knowledge calculus). This conceptual framework was extended to include a critical examination of the threshold for allowable risk in research involving children.[9] Allowable risk for such research is understood as that which falls within the bounds of discretion afforded to the parents as reasonable caretakers of their children. The subject of risk that may be undertaken by the observant Jew, as a reasonable caretaker of his body for G-d, is discussed in Section 4 of this book. A fascinating convergence in allowable risk in research between a duty-based approach and a rights-based approach is discussed in an appendix to Section 4 (available on the book's website), entitled "Participation in Clinical Research: Convergence of Jewish and Contemporary Perspectives."

As is evident from the discussion of Benjy's work leading to *Duty and Healing,* this book frames many of the subjects of his prior academic work within the context of Jewish law. As such, the book reveals the central influence of his faith, and its fundamental reliance on duties to others and to G-d, in earlier work on ethical problems. A central theme throughout Benjy's career was the elucidation of the obligations that govern the relationships among human beings, whether they be those found within the family or between the physician and her patient. Inasmuch as the book sheds light on deeper motivations in his earlier work, it also elucidates the nature of his faith. As evidenced by the central methodology of this book, Benjy's faith was one that was open to scrutiny by reason.

I believe that *Duty and Healing* will come to be regarded as Benjy's most important contribution to bioethics. Great works in bioethics don't merely give us a defensible answer to a particular moral problem; they change the way we see moral issues in general. Beauchamp and Childress's *Principles of Biomedical Ethics* framed moral problems as conflicts between ethical principles;[10] Pellegrino and Thomasma's *For the Patient's Good: The Restoration of Beneficence in Health Care* focused on central role of the virtuous moral agent;[11] and Jonsen and Toulmin's *The Abuse of Casuistry* saw moral reasoning as a process of appealing from the particulars of the case at hand to paradigmatic cases.[12] *Duty and Healing* adds yet another way of seeing moral problems, one in which individuals are set within a web of human relationships and obligations. As such, it is a welcome alternative to the thin description of the moral world offered by the language of rights that is so prevalent within our society. But this is better explained by Benjy than by me.

Debts of Gratitude

In the course of preparing this volume I have incurred many debts of gratitude. I could not have brought this book to completion without the help of the Freedman family and Gary Goldsand. Barbara Freedman ensured that the book remained true to both Benjy's project and the Jewish sources upon which it relies. Gary Goldsand, an exemplary doctoral candidate in religion and bioethics at the University of Toronto, assisted me throughout the editing process: We edited the text together, and he prepared the table of sources of Jewish law, glossary, and index for the book. Invaluable support and advice were provided by Heidi Freund (Routledge), Jim and Hilde Nelson (the academic editors of the series), Françoise Baylis, Kathleen Cranley Glass, Robert J. Levine, and colleagues at Mount Sinai Hospital in Toronto, particularly Theodore Freedman, Joseph Mapa, Alan Bernstein, and Rabbi Bernard Schulman.

Several of the sections in this book include parts of essays that have been previously published. I am grateful to the following organizations for permission to reprint Benjy's work here: the American Medical Association for part of "Offering truth: one ethical approach to the uninformed cancer patient," *Archives of Internal Medicine* 1993; 153: 572–576; the International Association of Physicians in AIDS Care for "Duty and healing: foundations of a Jewish bioethic (excerpt)," *Journal of the International Association of Physicians in AIDS Care* 1997; 3(3): 25–26, 45; and the Hastings Center for "Respectful service and reverent obedience," *Hastings Center Report* 1996; 26(4): 31–37.

Preparing this book for publication was a process filled with moments both happy and sad, and my partner of eight years, Anthony Belardo, stood by me through them all. That is, after all, the nature of the duty we owe each other, and its reward is the happiness we have found together.

My final words of gratitude must go to Benjamin Freedman. To him I owe not only my career, but also the fact that his moral example transfigured my rough countenance into something finer. It is a debt that only a lifetime of work and good deeds can repay.

Endnotes

1. Françoise Baylis, "Bioethics Scholar Remembered," *Canadian Medical Association Journal* 156 (1997): 1679; Françoise Baylis and Charles Weijer, "Remembering Benjamin Freedman (1951–1997)," *Hastings Center Report* 27, no. 3 (1997): 48; Trudo Lemmens, "Benjamin Freedman: A Life of Commitment," *NCBHR Communiqué* 8, no. 1 (1997): 6–7; Robert J. Levine, "Benjamin Freedman 1951–1997," *IRB: A Review of Human Subjects Research* 19, nos. 3, 4 (1997): 12; and Charles Weijer, "Duty and Healing: The Life Work of Benjamin Freedman," *Canadian Medical Association Journal* 156 (1997): 1553–1555.

2. Benjamin Freedman, "Competence, Marginal and Otherwise: Concepts and Ethics," *International Journal of Law and Psychiatry* 4 (1981): 53–72.

3. Benjamin Freedman, "A Moral Theory of Informed Consent," *Hastings Center Report* 5, no. 4 (1975): 32–39.

4. Benjamin Freedman, "On the Rights of the Voiceless," *Journal of Medicine and Philosophy* 3, no. 3 (1978): 196–210.

5. Benjamin Freedman, "Equipoise and the Ethics of Clinical Research," *New England Journal of Medicine* 317 (1987): 141–145.

6. Benjamin Freedman and Stanley H. Shapiro, "Ethics and Statistics in Clinical Research: Towards a More Comprehensive Examination," *Journal of Statistical Planning and Inference* 42 (1994): 223–240.

7. Benjamin Freedman, "Placebo-Controlled Trials and the Logic of Clinical Purpose," *IRB: A Review of Human Subjects Research* 12, no. 6 (1990): 1–6.

8. Benjamin Freedman, Abraham Fuks, and Charles Weijer, "Demarcating Research and Treatment: A Systematic Approach for the Analysis of the Ethics of Clinical Research," *Clinical Research* 40 (1992): 653–660.

9. Benjamin Freedman, Abraham Fuks, and Charles Weijer, "*In loco parentis:* Minimal Risk as an Ethical Threshold for Research Upon Children," *Hastings Center Report* 23, no. 2 (1993): 13–19.

10. T. L. Beauchamp and J. F. Childress, *Principles of Biomedical Ethics*, 4th ed. (New York: Oxford University Press, 1994).

11. E. D. Pelligrino and D. C. Thomasma, *For the Patient's Good: The*

Restoration of Beneficence in Health Care (New York: Oxford University Press, 1988).

12. A. Jonsen and S. Toulmin, *The Abuse of Casuistry* (Berkeley: University of California Press, 1988).

Goals and Framework

The Purposes of this Book

This is a book about certain personal moral questions that arise in the provision of medical treatment, especially of hospital care, and about one approach to reasoning about them. The book can be thought of as a religious project, for in it I try to explore Jewish texts and precedents and show different ways in which they may illuminate these issues. I intend the book to be a bioethical project as well, one that takes seriously the real world in which doctors practice and patients are treated and that suggests ways of improving our common understanding and resolution of those moral questions that arise in a health care context. It does this by marking the distinction between an ethics whose foundational language is duty, as is true of the Jewish approach, and contrasting that with our common Western ethical approach, whose basis is rights.

While actively seeking another model for understanding bioethical questions, I am reacting at the same time to a philosophical and bioethical approach that, in some fundamental ways, often misconstrues the moral reality felt by doctors, patients, and family members who deal with these ethical issues and to a Jewish literature that sometimes adopts a reductive and parochial stance to issues, one that fails to mobilize the extremely rich resources of Jewish legal and moral reasoning deposited over many centuries of inquiry.

A Typical Ethical Consultation

Let me give one example of what I mean, drawn from my records of hospital ethics consultations. Here and throughout this work, the consultation notes are taken from my own clinical consultative experience, in Canada and elsewhere. I prepare such notes, for my own records, following most requests in the hospital to meet to discuss the ethical issues underlying a particular case. They are available for review by the hospital ethics committee and are shared for educational purposes or otherwise at the request of the persons for whom the consult was performed. Names, location, and—in some cases—other identifying aspects of the cases have been removed or altered in the interests of confidentiality. In some cases, medical acronyms have been spelled out and explanations provided to assist the nonmedical reader. In all other respects, these consultation notes are unaltered.

ETHICS CONSULTATION: STEP BY STEP

Mrs. D is a ninety-two-year-old woman admitted to hospital in January after suffering a cerebrovascular accident [CVA; a major stroke, in which brain tissue is killed either by bleeding into the brain or by a loss of blood flow to the brain]. Presently she is on one of our long-term geriatric wards. She has had previous CVAs and minor strokes and is diagnosed as suffering from multi-infarct dementia, that is, a loss of cognitive abilities resulting from these strokes. She is therefore profoundly and permanently incapable of judging medical options and expressing choice amongst them. She has not prepared a living will, expressing how she would wish to be treated should she become incompetent, nor any other form of advance directive.

Two weeks ago, she developed serious pneumonia and high fever. Without the antibiotic treatment that was provided, she would almost certainly have died. She has been fed artificially by means of a naso-gastric [n-g] tube since admission; she has no gag reflex, and so cannot be fed orally. At present she is in reasonable condition except for dry gangrene of the toes. Mrs. D has minimal awareness; Dr. M felt she may acknowledge his presence, for example.

An incident precipitating the request for the consultation had occurred when the feeding tube came out and was being replaced. The daughter was present and became very upset at this intervention, and so the tube remained out for several days. Both the daughter and daughter-in-law have said that they wish to keep Mrs. D comfortable, and both have queried the aggressiveness of treatment. These two women are Mrs. D's closest relatives and main caregivers.

The issues at this point concerned withholding of treatment and of feeding. The members of the medical team were sympathetic to the family, but questioned whether the family's instructions do not amount to medical abandonment. We discussed at some length the issues and their common resolutions as they arise in the parallel case of persistent vegetative state [PVS], in which there is so much brain damage that patients lose the capacity for conscious experience. [Unlike coma, a state in which a patient is deeply unconscious, patients in PVS do have wake-sleep cycles—as often expressed, they are "awake but not aware."] In the case of a patient in PVS, we believe that the patient is beyond experiencing burdens or benefits. This can be taken as an argument for granting more weight to family decisions and sensitivities. It was, however, recognized that the level of awareness of Mrs. D takes her out of that class.

The fact that she is not in a persistent vegetative state cuts both ways in this case. On the one hand, it might argue in favor of prolonging life, for she, while deeply obtunded, is not devoid of all conscious experience. On the other hand, it could argue against feeding or other interventions that are capable of causing perceived discomfort. At times, while he was replacing the feeding tube, Dr. M felt that the patient was attempting to hold his hands back and that she was experiencing and expressing discomfort.

It was agreed that the family's wishes should be respected in this case, in which issues of values rather than those of medical appropriateness and feasibility are most prominent. It is possible, however, that the family protested the reinsertion of the feeding tube more out of a desire to experience some control over events than because they in fact wanted feeding stopped.

No discussion has been held with them as yet of other medical care choices to be made, for example, over the patient's resuscitation status [i.e., whether cardiopulmonary resuscitation ought to be attempted should Mrs D stop breathing, or her heart stop beating]. A comprehensive discussion about the patient's condition and available treatments should be held with them before further action is taken.

[Postscript: Several days following the consultation Dr. C told me that the patient had recovered a further degree of awareness. Efforts to sustain her nutritionally were being resumed, with the agreement of the family.]

Cases like this one are among the most common, and most difficult, ethical dilemmas faced in hospitals today for a number of reasons:

- The patient is incompetent, and so cannot tell us what she wants.
- The patient has not previously made her wishes known.
- The patient's quality of life, and especially her capacity for pleasurable experience, is low or absent.
- The decision implicates life or death.
- The decision to treat or not is dominated by ethical rather than technical considerations, since the "medical treatment" in question involves no high-tech, experimental apparatus. It is, simply, feeding.

Contemporary Secular and Jewish Understandings of Bioethical Issues

It is on these difficult yet common cases, if any, that writings on bioethics should be most illuminating, and it is in reaction to the ways in which they are commonly understood that this book was written, for writers on contemporary bioethics are apt to see them as raising the question of who has the *right* to decide. This is an important question of social ethics, one that deals with the adjudication of conflicting claims within society; by concentrating upon it, bioethics has made an important contribution. But ethical issues that arise within the clinical setting more commonly raise questions of personal ethics, questions that ask, from the moral actor's point of view: "What is the right thing to do?" As most commonly written today, bioethics assumes that its primary focus must be social ethics. But in trying to map ethical questions that arise in the hospital setting onto the particular concerns of social ethics, I believe, writers on bioethics totally misconstrue the ethical struggle that the parties to these ethical questions undergo, family members and doctors alike, and that is, "What does my personal or professional *duty* demand of me in this situation?"

Once such a dilemma hits the courtroom, to be sure, the lawyers for the various parties will undoubtedly frame the dispute as one over the rights of the family or of the medical staff. That, however, is the language of the law—our society's ultimate arbiter of social ethics— rather than of the moral genesis of the case, which lies in personal ethics. In the case of Mrs. D, for example, from their point of view, the family members of this patient intervened out of their personal moral duty to protect the patient. Correspondingly, the medical staff hesitated over obeying these family instructions because of their concern that this violates their professional moral duty to provide responsible and comprehensive patient care.

For their part, Jewish authors will characterize the issue as one of duty: May life-prolonging measures such as nutrition ever be withheld from a patient? Most Jewish authors, in denying this possibility, rely solely upon the medical facts of the case as construed by Jewish law, which values highly the prolongation of life (see Sections 2 and 4). This common, narrow focus upon the prolongation of life denies other Jewish values, however, and therefore cannot provide a comprehensive analysis of *halakha* [Jewish law]. It fails to notice, for example, that the involvement of the patient's daughter in this medical decision stems from her desire to fulfill her duty to honor her parent and that she faces here a dilemma: between providing nutrition to her mother and sparing her mother possible pain and definite indignity.

Secular and Jewish Approaches as Complementary

To a degree, the problems as well as the strengths associated with these two approaches may be seen as complementary. Secular bioethics, here and elsewhere, has a great deal to say about procedural questions—*who* will decide—but relatively less about substantive questions—*how* to decide. The success of secular bioethics at achieving consensus on social ethics, more often than not, involves approaches that are either directly or indirectly procedural. For example: The endorsement and analysis of the patient's right to informed consent, among the pillars of contemporary bioethics, is wholly derivative of the procedural resolve to allow competent patients to make their own medical decisions. By contrast, most current Jewish writers on bioethics concentrate almost exclusively upon substance—which decisions should be made and for what reason—and scarcely at all upon procedure.

If, as I believe, the basic strengths of the secular and Jewish approaches are so divergent, then perhaps as approaches they ought to be seen as complementary rather than contradictory, with each filling in for the other's deficiency. That, in large part, is the strategy that I adopt in this book. I try, for example, to show how the detailed modern philosophical discussions of informed consent are indeed of relevance to a Jewish view that requires that the individual patient serve as a responsible steward of his or her own body, an important procedural assignment largely ignored by Jewish writers to this date. By the same token, Jewish reflections on the nature of a person's responsibility to care for that body help supply one kind of answer to that perplexed patient who, granted the freedom that comes with the right to information, seeks moral guidance concerning how that freedom ought, substantively, to be exercised.

Methodological Choices in Jewish Bioethics

Secular and Jewish approaches to bioethics are not full parallels to one another. Secular bioethics is free to innovate new distinctions and approaches, or to adopt or adapt old ones, from a variety of normative traditions, provided these satisfy accepted principles of ethical reasoning. The rabbinic Jewish ethical and legal system is, by contrast, self-

contained, constrained by Divine scriptual rules and by precedents ac-
cumulated over thousands of years. This is not, of course, to say that
Jewish ethical and legal thinkers have not been influenced by their
surroundings and by the thought of their counterparts from other traditions. Outside influence may be overt or concealed; it may be expressed by borrowed or adapted ideas or by the vehement rejection of
an approach prominent among non-Jewish thinkers. None of this
negates the concept of Judaism as a self-contained normative system,
which requires that for an idea or approach to be validated it must be
derivable as a normative conclusion (whether or not originally derived
or suggested) from an acceptable *halakhic* source (including Scripture,
commentaries, accepted principles of legal reasoning, and so on). The
question is: Does this difference erect an insuperable barrier between
secular and Jewish approaches to bioethics?

The answer depends, I think, on the manner in which Jewish
sources are selected and by the methodology employed in interpreting
them. Jewish sources can be dealt with in ways that hermetically seal
them away from secular bioethical discourse. This is done through the
selection of sources and topics and by the way in which sources are interpreted and, through extrapolation, applied to broader circumstances. For, given the vast extent of Jewish sources that may be drawn
upon, and their complexity, some form of selection and interpretation
is an unavoidable necessity.

A writer may choose, for example, to concentrate upon such ritual
issues that arise in hospital practice as allowable violations of the laws
of the Sabbath, or rules regarding *tum'a* [impurity], and contact with
dead bodies. The concerns underlying these issues are foreign to a
modern readership, and their conclusions will only interest Jews already committed to rabbinic authority.

In this work, I have rather chosen to select Jewish legal sources
whose appeal is to reason (although almost always buttressed by Scripture), and which may be, for that reason, of more than parochial interest. In particular, I have chosen to concentrate upon those Jewish
sources that deal with *mitzvot bein adam l'chaveiro* [interpersonal
commandments] that have been relatively neglected in rabbinic discussions of the ethics of medical care.

I am myself an Orthodox Jew and am fully committed to that understanding of Judaism. In this work, however, I hope, by and large, to avoid those issues that serve to divide the streams of Judaism (Reform, Reconstructionist, Conservative, Orthodox, Chasidic, etc.). Those divisions have primarily arisen regarding matters of ritual law (*mitzvot bein adam lamakom*, commandments between man and G-d), rather than the laws governing interpersonal behavior.

I have also chosen to interpret those sources—or, more commonly, to adopt that traditional interpretation of those sources—in ways that speak most convincingly to the moral experience of patients and doctors, Jewish and gentile alike, as I have witnessed this in hospital work. While the need for selecting material is clear, an explicit choice of methodology may seem, from the viewpoint of traditional Judaism, more controversial, and even dangerous. Yet the difficulty and ambiguity of the texts that serve as the ultimate sources for rabbinic Jewish discussions—the Bible (the Written Law) and the Talmud (the Oral Law)—and the multiplicity of interpretations that have encrusted those texts make some choice of interpretation inevitable. When the text is irresolvably ambiguous, or when its interpretation has led to prolonged rabbinic controversy and dispute, I have simply chosen the approach that is of broader rational appeal.

Physicalism and the Choice of Methodology

To illustrate this point, let me give one example of a methodological choice I have exercised. The Talmud, as the starting point for Jewish legal discussion, couches its legal principles in concrete examples; the problem this poses is: How are those examples to be interpreted and, ultimately, extrapolated? For example, the Talmud will not speak of "the permissibility of medical treatment," in the abstract. It will instead speak of a specific practice thought at that time to be of medical benefit, such as bloodletting or the wearing of magical amulets, and discuss that practice's legal ramifications. Rather than state as a rule that a person is allowed to undergo occupational risk, the Talmud will speak of the fact that a man is allowed to climb a rickety ladder to pick fruit (see Section 4).

The question then becomes: How broadly should a concrete

example supplied by the Talmud be understood? Sometimes, rabbinic authorities interpret talmudic materials in a narrow way, which I term "physicalism." A physicalist approach is so called because it takes the physical characteristics of the concrete example the Talmud provides as the focus of interpretation and extrapolation, rather than more abstract principles underlying the example.

Consider the question of whether Jewish law permits a person to be a paid blood donor, inasmuch as persons have a religious obligation to avoid danger. Paid blood donation could quite simply fall under the abstract principle of allowed occupational risk and be allowed on that basis. The talmudic discussion that indicates that a person may climb a rickety ladder as part of the job is a good precedent from this point of view, although the concrete aspects of the analogy seem remote from the current case. (Climbing ladders does not resemble blood donation.) A "physicalist" approach might be taken instead: For example, a rabbi could rule it permissible on the basis that the Talmud's frequent references to bloodletting prove that, far from posing risk, it is a positive medical benefit![1] From the point of view of physicalism, blood donation bears a close resemblance to the early medical practice of bloodletting, while from the alternative focus upon underlying principle, which has been adopted in this work, the analogy is inapt. (Bloodletting was considered in the Talmud as of therapeutic benefit to the subject, while we consider blood donation to be a minor risk to the donor, rather than of therapeutic benefit.)

There is no question that either approach, or a combination of the two, represents acceptable methodology in *halakha*. The problem occurs when we attempt to convince others that what the *halakha* has said is worth listening to; for a "physicalist" interpretation of Jewish sources commits us not merely to talmudic ethical and legal reasoning, but to talmudic medical and scientific beliefs as well. In this work, therefore, as a methodological choice, I will consistently avoid "physicalist" understandings of Jewish sources.

The Scope of this Work

These choices imply that this work is not intended to present a comprehensive and final discussion of Jewish bioethics. When I subtitled this work *Foundations of a Jewish Bioethic,* I meant that quite literally. The problems dealt with are "foundational" in the sense that they cover only the essential elements that comprise health care ethics: Those are the ethics of medical choices made by competent persons (as described in the sections dealing with consent and with risk) and on behalf of incompetent persons (Section 1, "Family"), as well as the theory that allows us to distinguish competency from incompetency (Section 3).

The approach that I describe is, I think, but one approach to these issues, albeit one that has a substantial and sufficient basis in the relevant Jewish sources. I have tried to perform the modest task of describing "*a* Jewish bioethic." I do not try to cite every possible source, or to resolve every contradiction, in this work. It is not offered as the *only possible* Jewish approach to these issues, nor as the *most nearly correct* Jewish approach, nor, for that matter, as the one right, or most nearly correct, bioethical approach. It is offered for the consideration of any Jewish reader, from whichever religious stream, religiously committed or not, who is interested in seeing how Jewish sources and contemporary bioethical thought might creatively interact. It is offered, too, for the non-Jewish reader, as an example of how one tradition grounded in duty might approach problems of bioethics.

Trying to serve the needs of such a broad audience, with such diverse goals, is not a simple task. I have in this book tried to approach the task in stages. The first chapter is intended as a prologue. Taking as a specific example the current practice of hospital ethics consultation, I introduce the basic contrast between our currently most common bioethical approach, one that is grounded in rights and focuses upon social morality, and a Jewish approach to moral questions, one that speaks to personal as well as social ethics and whose basis is duty. This contrast is further elaborated in the heart of the book, which consists of four sections. Each of these describes one building block of this Jewish approach:

- *Section 1: Family* deals with the fundamental moral problem of the role of the family in reaching medical decisions for incompetent family members.

- *Section 2: Consent* introduces Jewish sources that imply that persons have a duty to care for their health, through seeking medical care and in other ways, and explains how such a duty requires, rather than precludes, the informed consent of patients.
- *Section 3: Competency* initiates an exploration of Jewish sources on the definition and implications of competency to consent to treatment and to fulfill other important social and ethical tasks.
- *Section 4: Risk* concludes the volume with a discussion of the substantive question of how Jewish law expects persons to arrive at decisions regarding medical care, consistent with their obligations to G-d and their fellows.

I intended the book to be read in the order presented. The later sections rest upon previous material. In addition, as the sections advance, I introduce progressively more Jewish sources, of increasing difficulty. Points of more specialized interest, as well as references, are presented in endnotes.

A more ambitious work than this would have covered many more topics and would have presented an extended exposition of Jewish sources. As it stands, this book is notably incomplete. Many topics of great interest in the rabbinic literature, such as truth-telling, the definition of death, and autopsies, have not been included. Issues that arise on a community level ("macro" and "meso" issues), such as the role of the hospital and the allocation of scarce resources, have also been excluded.

My focus throughout will be on the most common issues that arise on an individual level in medical treatment, those that all of us will face: as health care professionals, or as patients, or as the family members of patients. Yet even these issues are not treated comprehensively. Because I wish here to present the elements of a Jewish bioethic, I do not deal extensively with such complications as those that arise when these various elements come into conflict.

In summary, I have tried in this book to describe an ethic that places medical choices within the context of living a dutiful life. It was important, for that reason, that I present, in considerable detail, a number of cases of persons struggling with these choices. For the most part, I have tried to choose cases that illustrate the most common bioethical issues, rather than the most intricate or difficult issues, as this book is intended to do no more than provide the elements of a bioethical approach. I was constrained in my choice of cases by having restricted myself to those that actually were brought to me for the sake of consultation.

The reader should be aware that I do not believe that each resolution of the cases I describe is necessarily ideal, or even acceptable, as a matter of Jewish law. I describe the cases as I saw them, together with their results. As a clinical ethicist who works in a publicly supported hospital, I am obliged to respect my own professional constraints, both legal and ethical.

Transliteration

Hebrew words transliterated in the text are italicized. The transliteration used is simple, with the aim of enabling a non-Hebrew-speaker to approximate the Hebrew pronunciation of the term in question and a Hebrew-speaker to identify the word.

An ordained scholar and teacher of Judaism is known in English as "Rabbi," but his honorific is usually pronounced by Orthodox Jews as "Rav." I have throughout used the prefix *R* to signify ordination; thus, for example, R Moshe Feinstein would be read, "Rav Moshe Feinstein."

Pronunciation Key

Vowels:

a as in "calm"; *e* as in "egg"; *i* as in "hid" or as in "piece"; *o* as in "hold"; *u* as in "huge"; *ai* as in "tie"; *ei* as in "weigh."

Consonants:

All consonants are pronounced "hard," for example, *c* as in "car," not "pace." *ch* and *kh* represent the Hebrew letters *chet* and *khaf*, respectively. Most contemporary Hebrew-speakers pronounce them in identical guttural fashion, as in the Scottish "loch."

The apostrophe is used to differentiate vowels that are pronounced separately; for exapmle, *Ra'avad* is pronounced "Ra-a-vad."

Sources: Translation and Citation

Translations

All translations used in the text are my own. (For that reason, in those cases where an unusual translation is used, I include the Hebrew original in transliteration.) I have tried in translating material to remain as close to the letter of the original as possible, for the sake of "flavor" as well as of accuracy. Some deviations were unavoidable, however. Up until the time of compilation of the Talmud and in some cases beyond (e.g., *midrashim*), the texts are unpunctuated; all punctuation supplied is therefore that which fits my own understanding of the texts in question. Other minor deviations were done for stylistic reasons. Stock phrases, such as the Divine epithet "the Holy One, Blessed Be He"—themselves commonly abbreviated in rabbinic literature—I usually render in short form, as (in the case of this particular epithet) "the Holy One."

The reader may not find these texts easy to read. The fault is not entirely that of the translator. Rabbinic texts, and especially discussions from the Talmud, are very difficult to follow even for those completely familiar with the language. I have occasionally interpolated in square brackets—[ ]—explanatory remarks. These are always my own, unless otherwise indicated or cited. The most common of these exceptions is the bracketed inclusion of explanations of the text of the Babylonian Talmud offered by Rashi (the acronym of the early medieval French rabbi R Shlomo Yitzchaki), who was by far the most influential commentator upon the Talmud.

The forms of reference and citation I use are those common to contemporary students of Jewish tradition, as described here.

Sources of Jewish Law and Normative Thought

Sources used here include: the books of the Bible accepted into the Jewish canon. Biblical citations are given using the common English names of the books and are presented by chapter and verse (separated by a period), corresponding to the traditional Jewish (Masoretic) division of the Bible. Thus, 2 Kings 12.4 refers to the second book of Kings (known in Hebrew as *M'lakhim Beit*), twelfth chapter, fourth verse.

A further source is the Mishna, a compilation of rabbinic legal rulings whose editing was completed by the year 200 CE. (Material from this period and of the same nature that was not included within the Mishna is known as *b'raita,* plural *b'raitot.*) The Gemara is a compilation of rabbinic discussions all of which originate with questions associated with the interpretation of the Mishna (but by no means ending with that). Talmud refers to the combination of Mishna and Gemara. We have in our possession two such collections: the *Talmud Bavli* (signified in this text by the abbreviation TB), or Babylonian Talmud, most of which was collected and edited by the conclusion of the fifth century of the common era; and the earlier compilation, the *Talmud Yerushalmi* (abbreviated TY), the Jerusalem (or Palestinian) Talmud. The *Talmud Bavli* is the lengthier of the two, and (in cases of conflict) is generally the more authoritative.

The Babylonian Talmud is divided into volumes known as tractates, and is cited by a double-sided folio page corresponding to a standard print presentation. Thus, TB *Sanhedrin* 84a refers to the first side of page 84 in the tractate Sanhedrin of the Babylonian Talmud. The Jerusalem Talmud is sometimes cited by reference to standard pagination as well, but more usually (and loosely) is cited by tractate, chapter, and chapter subdivision (known as *halakha,* law). Thus, TY *K'tubot* 3.4 refers to the third chapter and fourth *halakha* of the Jerusalem Talmud's tractate *K'tubot.*

The many commentaries on the Talmud—the most important of which are by Rashi, noted earlier, and by those commentators who followed Rashi in France and Germany, whose work is collected under the name *Tosfot* (additions)—are ordinarily arranged according to the talmudic pagination; *Tosfot* commenting upon TB *Sanhedrin* 84a would be cited as *Tosfot* TB *Sanhedrin* 84a and would be found on that folio in the standard (Romm) edition. When it is uncertain which of *Tosfot's* comments there is being referred to, I specify the talmudic words (s.v.—Latin: *sub verbum*) that the commentator is discussing; thus "s.v. *v'hinei*" is the comment on the word *v'hinei* in the text.

There are two main codifications of Jewish law to which I will refer. The earlier is the *Mishne Tora* of Rambam (the acronym of R Moshe ben Maimon, Maimonides, 1135–1204, who worked in Spain and Egypt). While divided into fourteen "books," it is usually referenced by chapter and section within thematic subdivisions of those books (leaving the discovery of which book the subdivision is to be found in as an exercise for the student). Thus, Rambam, *Hilkhot Mamrim* 6.10 refers to the tenth section of the sixth chapter of *Hilkhot Mamrim* in the *Mishne Tora*. (When referring to other works of Rambam the title is cited.) The other major compilation is that of R Yosef Karo (1488–1575), the *Shulchan Arukh*. It (as well as its predecessor, the *Tur Shulchan Arukh*) is split into four main thematic divisions and is subdivided into sections and subsections. Thus, *Yore Dei'a* 339.2 refers to the division *Yore Dei'a*, section 339, paragraph 2. Commentaries to both of these codes are generally referenced to the text on which they comment, as was true of commentators upon the Talmud.

The other main source material upon which I draw is the responsa (singular: *responsum*) literature, compilations of responses the rabbinic author of the work had provided to questions posed of him regarding Jewish law. Since the early medieval period, this literature has been the main source for detailed rabbinic discussion and innovation, and cumulatively represents many thousands of volumes of such work. Some, but not all, of the responsa authors arranged their work according to the four divisions of the *Shulchan Arukh,* and some of these single-author collections have run to many volumes. Within each volume, the internal division is generally done by section; usually each section refers to a different question that has been posed. These sections may in turn be subdivided further. Thus R Moshe Feinstein, Responsa *Igrot Moshe, Choshen Mishpat,* 2, Section 63, s.v. *'al kol panim keivan* refers to Rav Moshe Feinstein's second volume of responsa dealing with questions associated with the division of the *Shulchan Arukh* known as *Choshen Mishpat;* more specifically, with the sixty-third section (or "question"), in the subsection beginning with the words *'al kol panim keivan.*

A variety of other Jewish sources—rabbinic volumes, commentaries upon the Bible (including *midrashim*), the Zohar, and many others—have been utilized, as well as scholarly material in medicine, bioethics, Jewish bioethics, and so on. Rather than cram all of this into a Procrustean endnote style, I have tried in each case to use the citation format that would be most recognizable to the sort of person likely to look that citation up.

Until the age of computerization, to identify responsa dealing with some particular question or other was extremely difficult. The material was uncatalogued and unindexed, and the student's choices were to either read everything every rabbi had ever written or speak to someone who had (and who remembers it all). Bar-Ilan University's Responsa Project, a computerized full-text database that includes hundreds of responsa volumes as well as the other chief sources of Jewish law in fully searchable form (and on a single CD!), has transformed that situation. Without that single shiny disk in my computer, the present work would probably never have come to pass.

Acknowledgments

I have incurred a number of debts of gratitude over the development of this manuscript. My wife, Barbara, read and commented upon the entire manuscript and provided encouragement, numerous suggestions, and a degree of grounding in the priorities of reality. My older children, Ariela, Orit, and Avidan, and my son-in-law, Jeremy Wexler, each read and commented upon portions of the work; my youngest son, Menachem, contributed in other ways. Some of my colleagues at McGill were also helpful; I would like to single out Kathy Glass, Charles Weijer, and Carl Elliott. Special thanks is owed to Karen Lebacqz, who provided detailed comments based on a close and sympathetic, but critical, reading. John Kleinig, of John Jay College/CUNY, helped with some issues in early drafts of some material. Shimon Glick, of Israel's Ben-Gurion University of the Negev, provided numerous useful suggestions and pointed me to some important sources and references.

Support and encouragement has always been provided to me by

colleagues—doctors, nurses, social workers, and other personnel—at the Sir Mortimer B. Davis Jewish General Hospital of Montreal; without their help, I would not have begun this work and could not have completed it. I would like to particularly thank Drs. Harold Frank, Paul Heilpern, Andre Dascal, and Jack Mendelson and Messrs. Archie Deskin and Henri Elbaz. Dr. Perle Feldman and Dr. Ronnie Schondorf also provided useful input to the manuscript.

Portions of this manuscript, and the arguments presented here, were included in presentations given at the Fifth World Congress on AIDS, Montreal, June 7, 1989; at Albert Einstein Medical Center (of Philadelphia), October 22–24, 1990; at the Canadian Bioethics Society, Quebec City, November 23, 1990; at Liberal Arts College, Concordia University, Montreal, March 14, 1991; at Brown University, April 17, 1991; at the Society for Bioethics Consultation, Toronto, September 5, 1991; at the 4th International Congress on Ethics in Medicine, October 16, 1991, Jerusalem, Israel; at the YMHA Winnipeg, February 18, 1992; at the Rabbinic Council of Montreal, Dollard-des-Ormeaux, Quebec, March 26, 1992; at Albert Einstein College of Medicine, Bronx, New York, April 9, 1992; at Lillian Burden Jewish Community Annual Memorial Lecture, London, Ontario, September 16, 1992; at the Canadian Society of Bioethics, Montreal, November 18, 1993; at Jakobovits Centre for Jewish Medical Ethics, Beersheba, Israel, July 28, 1994; and at the Mesorah Society (in association with the American Psychiatric Association), Miami, May 23, 1995; as well as on a number of occasions at McGill University and the Sir Mortimer B. Davis Jewish General Hospital of Montreal. I am grateful for comments and suggestions made by other speakers and members of the audience on these occasions.

In the traditional phrase, "From all my teachers have I learned; and from my colleagues, even more than from them; and from my students, even more than from them."[2] For this work, I need to add, "and from our patients and their families, even more than from them." The opportunity to speak with persons struggling with the most intimate questions of meaning in life and in death is a great privilege, for which I am most grateful.

This book is dedicated to Barbara, Ariela, Orit, Avidan, and Menachem, and it is consecrated to my mother, Anne z'l; to my father, Manuel z'l; and to my brother Gary z'l.

Endnotes

1. See R Moshe Feinstein, *Responsa Igrot Moshe, Choshen Mishpat,* 1, 103.*

2. TB *Ta'anit* 7a.

Duty and Clinical Ethics Consultations from a Jewish Viewpoint

Introduction

Clinical ethical consultation is, in many respects, a practice done by, at, and for the margin. The practice of such consultations began very recently. Its practitioners come from a diverse group of backgrounds with highly disparate qualifications and are employed in a variety of settings with very different expectations. Even in those institutions where clinical ethics consultation has been most firmly and longest established, it remains highly unusual for a case to become the subject of a formal ethics consultation.

Clinical Ethics Consultations

For these very reasons clinical ethics consultation deserves close examination. Consultants work around the edges of the health care team, with respect to cases that are themselves out of the ordinary. These cases, and the contribution to their resolution that can come from clinical ethics consultants, challenge us to reexamine our understanding of what kinds of ethical problems exist in health care, of how they arise, and of how they can be resolved. For this same reason, clinical ethics consultations provide a useful context for understanding some ways in which a Jewish approach may differ from our current bioethical approaches.

I want now to consider the practice of clinical ethics consultation. What are its philosophical underpinnings? What are the goals of a consultation? What does it mean, for example, to say that a consultation has succeeded? For that matter: What does it mean to hold an ethics consultation? When somebody—who?—asks for a consultation, and somebody—how?—responds to that request, what has been done? And how is it to be judged? And when should it be done, when completed, and how improved?

A theoretical framework is needed for this inquiry. For the sake of clarity, I will speak of three different theoretical approaches to ethical consultation. As theoretical constructs, each of these represents an ideal type. Many writers merge elements of two or three of these models—those who work in clinical ethics tend to theoretical eclecticism—and while some incline more clearly to one model, none that I know of reflects any one of these models in its complete and pure form. That does not mean that the models are "straw men," set up to be knocked down, any more than is any other unrealistically simple thought experiment (e.g., of motion in a frictionless world) pursued for the sake of clarification. And theory does matter, even in the practical world of ethical consultants. Theory can set the initial conditions, desiderata, and background understanding of consultations. As I will try to show later, this may be done subtly enough that they are never even recognized as theoretical choices.

In one view, the job of consultants is grounded in rights: The consultant should discover what rights are at issue, whether they conflict, and how this conflict may be resolved. Most naturally, in this view, the consultant's primary task is procedural: to discover who has the right to decide an ethical issue and to preserve that person's autonomy. Another view has it that ethics serves, like other consultative specialty services, as assistance to a perplexed decision maker; this view emphasizes prerogative and status. I shall explore a third view, centering about duty and nurtured by Jewish sources.[1]

Consultation in Practice: One Case

Hospital-based clinical ethical consultation has grown explosively in the past ten years. One important attraction of clinical ethics has been its practical side, the promise it holds out that what began as quite abstract philosophizing may positively affect the resolution of a case. This practical bent binds the various views about ethics consultation. Each of these views, in its own way, has something to say about how ethics consultation should be done and how ethics consultants (and their clients) should understand this process. Each has a claim to understanding and evaluating the clinical ethics consultation. But for each, the starting point is the case itself. Following is one such case.

ETHICS CONSULTATON: LET ME DIE

The consultation, requested by Dr. G, concerned his ninety-eight-year-old patient, Mrs. T, who had been admitted to the hospital with congestive heart failure and pneumonia. For a woman of her years, she had maintained remarkably good health, apart from urinary incontinence of many years' standing and more recent mild bowel incontinence. The precipitating cause of the consultation: Mrs. T's statement "I am just tired; let me die a natural death." She has repeated this desire to Dr. G for the last four days running.

The patient continues to be a very sharp and lucid woman, although she is blind and nearly deaf. To illustrate the kind of woman she is, Dr. G told me how she had traveled to Florida when she was well into her eighties in order to care for her daughter, who was dying of cancer.

Mrs. T maintains a close relationship with her family, including a son, daughter-in-law, and granddaughter. They come to visit frequently; until her admission they had been caring for Mrs. T well, enabling her to maintain her own apartment. Dr. G had not spoken to them about Mrs. T's desire, pending the opportunity to speak with me; he does not, therefore, know their feelings about this.

Dr. G, a family physician who is managing her hospital care, has been Mrs. T's primary physician for about twenty years. He feels terrible ambivalence about agreeing to her wish to withdraw treatment, and anguish is evident on his face as he asks: "Is this my decision to make or hers? Isn't she asking me to exercise more power than any human being should have?"

In the course of our discussion I probed a number of areas

that often underlie a patient's wish to withdraw treatment. Did Mrs. T feel as though she is a burden upon others? Was there some inadequacy in care that might be rectified, making her change her mind—some neglect of nursing care, some mindless, bureaucratically inspired indignity? The answer was no: Her support systems have held up well; her request is something she is asking for herself, although she knows her family will miss her. Her debilitated condition is not likely to improve despite treatment, particularly because she has been refusing physiotherapy and has not been mobilized.

The case Dr. G presented seemed inescapably to lead toward respecting her wishes by withdrawing those treatments being provided to prolong her life (while maintaining those needed for Mrs. T's comfort). She was not, in his judgment, clinically depressed; he feels no need for a consultation from the psychiatry service, and she would be insulted if he suggested this to her.

I suggested one final approach he might try. It remains possible that Mrs. T was refusing treatment not so she might die, but rather as a final means of asserting control over her own life and destiny. Blind, deaf, bedridden, utterly dependent upon others, her only effective means of acting might be to say no. Perhaps, were she given an alternative realm of decision making, she could reconsider her global refusal. One way of doing this would be for Dr. G to discuss with Mrs. T her critical intervention status—decisions about cardiac and pulmonary resuscitation, and her choices about pain medication, intravenous, and so forth.

Both Dr. G and I knew there was little scope for choice about these matters. Given her underlying heart condition, once her heart stops it will be impossible to start it again (not to mention the fact that any effort at heart massage will immediately splinter this ninety-eight-year-old woman's rib cage). Nonetheless, he felt she was certainly lucid enough and interested enough in her condition to handle such a discussion. If all she needs is an assurance that she retains mastery of her fate, such a discussion might satisfy that demand.

Dr. G reported back to me after speaking with Mrs. T. She appreciated his concern and willingness to spend this time with her, and told him she certainly did not wish to be resuscitated should her heart stop or should she stop breathing. At the same time, though, she told Dr. G she wanted all other treatments stopped as well, except for those keeping her comfortable. Her wishes were respected. She died very shortly thereafter, of heart failure.

The Model of Rights

Bioethics and the Patients' Rights Movement

The patients' rights movement was a powerful, perhaps dominant, motivating force behind the development of contemporary bioethics. A number of streams fed what became a swift current: concern over unethical human research, particularly that conducted upon vulnerable populations; perceived abuses of psychiatry; general distrust of expertise and authority figures in the established social hierarchy of power.

A view of clinical ethics consultation as primarily concerned with rights flows from this understanding of the underpinnings of the bioethics movement. Within this understanding, hospitals are seen as places in which the rights of patients are poorly articulated, rarely acknowledged, and commonly violated. An early academic, judicial, and legislative task was the establishment and description of these rights. At that stage, discussion focused upon the psychiatric patient's right to treatment (soon to be followed by the patient's right to refuse treatment); the right of informed consent to treatment and to research; the right to require that unwanted treatment be withheld or withdrawn, a right that could also be exercised prospectively (in the form of a living will or advance directive); and rights to control the dissemination of medical information, that is, to protection of medical confidences, among many others.

The clinical ethics consultation can be seen as the second stage in this development. Armed with an expanded and revitalized understanding of the rights of patients, the ethics consultant can serve to clarify and often help resolve moral issues that arise within the hospital, for in this view, those issues involve the failure to respect rights. To be sure, patients' rights will not be enough for this purpose. In some cases, patients will claim positive rights, rights to be provided with some good or service. These positive rights may collide with scarce hospital resources, and therefore with the equal positive claim of other patients. In some cases, that is, one patient's rights may conflict with those of another. Moreover, other persons within the setting—notably (although not exclusively) physicians, nurses, and other health care providers—possess rights as well. In addition to vindicating the rights of patients, then, the job of clinical ethics consultant becomes one of helping to understand and, perhaps, reconcile conflicting claims of rights.[2]

Ethics Consultations Within the Model of Rights:
Social Ethics and Conflict

True to its roots, this view of hospital ethics consultation would be restricted to what I have called, in my Introduction, social ethics, the adjudication of conflicting demands made by persons within society. These claims are expressed in terms of rights, which therefore act as the primary (or primordial) ethical concept in play. Other ethical concepts that may be introduced into the discussion are secondary to rights. Duties, for example, are created by rights; for instance, my duty to treat the patient is secondary to the patient's right (under specified circumstances) to be treated.

How would this rights-centered view understand a clinical ethics consultation? Ethical issues manifest as conflict. A right is at risk, either because it may be violated or because two rights claims are colliding. Therefore, the consultation is forced to focus upon defined, narrow issues: What does the right require? Whose rights supersede? The possible outcomes of the consultation are similarly predefined as one of two polar choices. Someone will win, and in winning—because the genesis of the consultation was conflict—someone else must lose. For this view, the role of the consultant is to pick the winner. Within our society, at once so fascinated by the substance of legal issues and so repulsed by the enormous resources consumed by the legal process, some version of this model of ethics consultation as rights adjudication is inevitably attractive: It is the justice of the courtroom, without the courtroom.

The rights model of consultation, or any alternative model, provides a particular understanding of how ethics consultation can and should proceed—a job description, if you like. As such, it could be neither proved nor disproved, any more than can baking or candlestick making. Insofar as all these models offer competing visions of how to respond to felt ethical issues within the clinical setting, however, it is fair to judge them by different kinds of criteria; for example, do they provide novel and useful insight into these ethical issues? While no model will bind an ethics consultant in practice, theoretical constructs do suggest a framework within which a proposed ethical discussion may be held. It is therefore fair to ask how an ethics consultant using a version of the rights model would have reacted to the case of Dr. G and Mrs. T.

No case could be more straightforward than this one, from the point of view of one adhering to the rights model. That Mrs. T is a competent adult is undisputed. She has the right to refuse any and all medical interventions. There is no conflict of rights here; Dr. G has no right to perpetrate medical treatment without his patient's consent. This is true whether the patient is eighteen or ninety-eight, whether the medical interventions in question are benign and effective or, as here, are likely doomed to failure. And that is all there is to be said. The suggestions I tried out on Dr. G are quite beside the point of the consultation and are mere delaying tactics, although the delay they entail may not be harmful (that is, seriously in violation of the patient's rights).

The only puzzle posed by the case from the rights point of view may be the fact that it was brought up at all, since the issue was so clear. But that puzzle quickly dissipates. Dr. G was a physician of many years' practice, acculturated to medicine in the bad old days when patients' rights were misunderstood, ignored, or violated.

Do Typical Consultations Involve Conflicts of Rights?

There is reason to think that the rights approach would not have been helpful in this very typical case, that indeed, at a fundamental level, it misunderstands the nature of what was at stake. For the consultation requested by Dr. G was predicated not upon conflict, but upon uncertainty. In a sense, Dr. G had hesitated to do what (arguably) was necessitated by respect for Mrs. T's rights. But this was not because he was unaware of her right to refuse treatment, as a legal and intellectual matter: Elderly or not, Dr. G could still read. Nor was he refusing to act in compliance with her rights; had that been so, he never would have requested the consultation.

A conflict of rights presupposes two persons assertively demanding that their contrary desires be respected. There was none of that here, either. Dr. G did not speak the language of power, of authority, of rights as trumps—or as clubs. He was, rather, hesitant, uncertain, ambivalent, and conflicted. He did not need someone to tell him what the rights of the patient demand of him. What he sought was a way to live conscientiously within the world of his profession, true to long-standing commitments.

The fact that a model of rights would not have been helpful to Dr. G is not, of course, the end of the story. Another question remains: Would the model have been helpful to Mrs. T? I can only speculate. Although I rarely do a consultation without speaking with the patient (or, if incompetent, the patient's family), I did not speak with Mrs. T. The reason: As I came to understand the issue, it did not concern Mrs. T's care—ultimately, I believed, her wishes would be respected—but rather how Dr. G would come to that point. Yet without speaking to Mrs. T, I have spoken to many Mrs. T's. Would she have expected or wanted me to explain the model of rights to Dr. G? I doubt it. Recall that these two had a relationship lasting over twenty years. It seems to me improbable that Mrs. T would have chosen to short-circuit the difficult process Dr. G faced of letting her go by a bare assertion that such is her right. Had that been what she wanted, she would have had obvious recourse to the law itself. (And in general, the model of rights faces the objection that by its own lights it is in many ways just a pale imitation of what these issues really need, namely, a lawsuit.)

Was this case really an occasion for an ethics consultation? After such a case, an ethics consultant will often say something like, "It was no big ethical deal" or "That wasn't really philosophy" or "It was really more like social work, or hand-holding." For the rights model, these cases are so cut-and-dried, so devoid of interest, as to be relegated to the periphery of ethics consultation. In a well-ordered world, with physicians receiving proper training in patients' rights, they would vanish. It is worth pointing out that in my own experience, and that of every clinical ethics consultant I have ever spoken to, cases like that of Dr. G, which center around questions of personal morality, are overwhelmingly more common than those posing gritty social ethical questions of irreconcilable conflict. One central task for a model of consultation is the provision of perspective, and in this the model of rights seems to me notably lacking: It places at the periphery those cases that experience shows constitute the core of ethics consultations.

The Model of Expert Counselor

Ethics as a Consultative Specialty

Partly as a reaction to the early ethics literature's focus upon rights, and bolstered by the institutionalization and acculturation of bioethics within clinical settings, another model has been fostered. Consider the following representative statements. As earlier, in delineating the model of expert counselor I intend to describe an ideal type. The authors of the following quotations obviously incline toward the model of expert consultation, but none of them embraces *tout court* the pure model as it is described here.

> It is not the function of the ethics consultant to deliver "right answers" to the moral quandaries of physicians. . . . Since justified norms of behavior are socially produced outcomes, the ethics consultant cannot claim to know what is morally right independently of participation by others in the investigative process. . . . [T]hus, the consulting ethicist . . . may provide informed recommendations for consideration by the physician consulted.[3]

No one profession has a corner on eternal ethical truths. If the physician is the professional who is primarily responsible for the patient, a medical ethicist with insight provided by the literary disciplines can offer help but cannot take over decision making or presume to tell the physician what to do. . . . [T]here will certainly be situations in which the ethicist advocates one opinion over another, but he or she should only perform this service when asked and should do so without appearing to take charge of decision making or assuming an air of infallibility.[4]

In this model, the ethicist acts as an expert counselor to those who face unusually difficult ethical choices. Almost inevitably in this model, the client of the consultation is a treating physician, and the focus of the consultation is a choice the physician confronts. For this reason, as in the model of rights, the typical consultation revolves around conflict: diverse, irreconcilable choices. However, for the expert consultation model the conflict need not involve persons and their irreconcilable claims of right, but rather actions and their various associated risks, costs, and benefits.

The goal of the consultation is to be helpful to the physician who requested it, by elucidating the ethical issue confronted, exploring alternatives, sharing perspectives drawn from the literature or approaches to the issue taken elsewhere, and so forth. Just as is true of medical consultations—for example, an infectious-disease specialist consulting at the request of the patient's primary-care physician—the final decision remains in the hands of the physician requesting the consultation.

In a number of versions, the model of the expert counselor is gaining force. It has certainly been found congenial within the clinical setting and is attractively nonthreatening to physicians, whose voice is usually dominant in hiring hospital-based ethicists. As before, however, the question to be asked is whether the model is helpful. Would it provide a useful and fruitful way of understanding the clinical ethics consultation?

Who Owns an Ethical Problem?
Problems of Identification and Perspective

The first point that must be made is that the focus this model tends to put upon the physician as decision maker seems strangely anachronistic within the usual setting of ethics consultation, namely, the hospital. Most clinical ethics consultations revolve around a patient's treatment. (In this way the case of Dr. G and Mrs. T was atypical, as explained earlier.) Hospital treatment is not provided by "the doctor," but rather by a slew of persons: senior physicians responsible for coordinating care, consultants, medical students and residents in various stages of training, nurses, therapists of various kinds, ward clerks, orderlies—this list is far from complete. Quite often, the patient is a moveable feast for whole regions of the hospital, transferred from emergency to surgery to infectious disease to geriatrics. This is not a mob of bystanders to "the doctor" treating the patient— whichever treating physician happens, for whatever reason, to be singled out as "the doctor." Each has a role to play, which can be done well or poorly. The conduct of each will affect the patient's status and recovery, and the choices of one particular doctor should not be understood as primary and ultimate.

Granting "the doctor" the central and privileged role, as authors tending toward this model do, misreads the facts of contemporary hospital care and may result in very damaging deformations of the consultation process. It narrows the scope of questions that may be asked in a consultation and information that may be sought. Kenneth Simpson's practice shows this characteristic: "Only the attending physician can request an ethics consultation, and access to the patient or members of the patient's family depends on the attending physician's consent."[5] Whether these restrictions are exercised or not, they profoundly undermine the credibility of each consultation, just as there is never any reason to believe a newspaper whose contents must be approved by the state before publication. And so I believe that hospitals rarely, if ever, begin an ethics consultation service motivated primarily by the desire to counsel their perplexed physicians; if they do, they certainly don't advertise that fact.

But if this model of expert consultancy to troubled physicians makes little sense as the sole, or even main, model of consultation, does it not make sense as one task a consultant may face? For example, does it not fairly represent the consultation held with Dr. G? Although that consultation ended that way, I think the model misrepresents the terms under which it began, and here we come to the crux of the difficulty with this model, the vacuum that lurks at its center.

As I read him, Dr. G was not primarily interested in ethical psychotherapy or values clarification. He wanted to know what might have been overlooked (an allowable intervention within the consultative model), but he also wanted to know if what he was thinking and how he was acting were wrong. He wanted to speak to me because he trusted my knowledge and training (again, allowable motives in the consultation model), but also because he respected my own judgment and integrity. He would have had, I think, no interest in speaking to an ethical cipher. In short: He wanted to do right by his patient, and he wanted to know what I thought that might involve. He did not ask to speak with me so that he could be told, "This is what you think is right in this case; this is what your values dictate." But given the nature of this model, that is how each consultation is foreordained to conclude—unless, of course, the pragmatic inclination of ethics consultants steps in to relax the theoretical rigor of neutrality, to suspend, that is, this model.

Can the model be saved? The most obvious modification, given what was said earlier, would be to broaden the scope of those for whom consultation may be provided, in recognition of the fact that it is not just "the doctor" who faces bioethical issues. This is the stance of Pellegrino, Siegler, and Singer:

> The ethicist's aim should be to enable, empower, and enhance the decision-making capabilities of patient, doctor, and family. The ethicist should not make the decision for them, or worse still, impose his or her ethical values or beliefs on the primary decision makers.[6]

This is certainly a step in the right direction. The goals of enabling and empowering all of the various actors in the bioethical drama are often necessary. Yet the problem just noted remains. At the close of discussion, all that has been done is the clarification of a concatenated variety of points of view: "This is what *you* think is right; and you; and you . . ."

It is common, even usual, for a consultation to end with no change in the treatment plan, or in the bottom-line views of the participants. Those consultations are seen as valuable when and because the participants feel that their initial sense of the situation has been validated. Validation, however, implies external assessment and evaluation. If the goal of the consultation was purely that of clarification, the participants are fooling themselves in feeling validated, for all the consultation has done is hold up their initial ethical views before a clean and well-lighted mirror.

Before leaving this model, there is one final problem to note. Such a consultation, ending with "This is what you—and you, and you—think," particularizes the ethical views of the participants, and thereby misrepresents them. For participants in these consultations—providers, patients, and family alike—not only have views, but have views *about a particular issue:* the proper treatment of a patient. They are all talking about the same thing; if they are in conflict, they are all in conflict about the same thing. This unifying factor, the common concern for the good of the patient, is splintered in a consultation process that sees its task as facilitating decision makers, rather than decisions.

The Model of Duty

In one sense, it is not surprising that the model of duty has received so little attention.[7] The model of expert consultation trades upon a traditional and still-powerful professional hierarchy; that of rights, our common, largely procedural, approach to social ethics. By contrast, we have no public shared understanding of duties and personal morality. We indeed pride ourselves upon developing a legal system that maintains personal morality apart from public discourse, as a private preserve.

Typical Consultations: Clarifying Rights or Duties?

Yet in another sense, this is very surprising indeed, for in my experience, at any rate, the claims and dilemmas of duty suffuse the consultative experience. Consultations within the clinical setting do not, after all, occur within a fully public setting; a consult is not a trial. In this respect, too, consultations occur at the margin: the borderline between the utterly private and the absolutely public. Within the normative universe of the consultation, I find, although the particulars may be in dispute, the claims of duty in general are deeply respected. The family has one view, the doctor another. At the same time, each recognizes the ethical basis of the other's stance.

Any theory of duty is ultimately substantive, not structural. To understand duty fully, a particular theory detailing duties must be provided, and the theory I shall use for that purpose in this book is duty as understood from Jewish sources. I shall describe a nonparochial Jewish understanding that has much to commend itself on its own merits to those with no commitment to the Jewish tradition per se. As we approach this substantive view, however, we need to get more clear about what grounding an ethics consultation in duty implies.

It is true that clinical ethics consultations are sometimes requested as an approach to solving an underlying problem that is not ethical in nature: for example, as a final ploy to assuage a disgruntled family member in an effort to avert threatened legal action or as a means for opening communication amongst health care providers within a troubled neonatal intensive care unit. Arguably, if in these cases the ethics consultants can perform a useful function, they should agree to do so. But these are not the purposes of ethics consultations.

In their pure form, consultations begin with a question of duty. I have argued that Dr. G was not concerned with his rights, or with those of Mrs. T. My further claim that he was not asking for a consultation to clarify his own options and views may have been more opaque, for he did in a way want such clarification: not, however, because he wanted to know what he would think—in a calm, clarified, and reflective moment—was the right thing to do, but because he wanted to know what *was* the right thing to do, or, better yet, *whether there was* a right thing to do here.

Duty Toward the Patient
as the Ethical Common Denominator

If there is a single duty that is the glue holding together ethics consultations that begin in conflict, it is the duty to seek the right course of action in treating the patient. Consider the following excerpt from a consultation.[8]

ETHICS CONSULTATION: AN OFFER OF TRUTH

Mrs. A is a woman in her sixties with colon cancer that has caused metastatic liver involvement and a mass in the abdomen. She is not expected to survive more than a few weeks. Other than a course of antibiotics, which she was just about to complete, no active treatment is indicated or intended. She is alert. She knows that she has an infection; her family refuses to inform her that she has cancer. The precipitating cause of the ethical consultation, requested by the newly assigned treating physician (Dr. H), is his ethical discomfort with treating Mrs. A in this manner.

As clinical ethicist, I met with Dr. H and the involved members of the patient's family (husband, daughter, son). Most of the discussion was held with the son; the husband, a first-generation Greek-Canadian immigrant, speaks little English and was at any rate somewhat withdrawn. As I expected, they are a close family, deeply solicitous of the patient, and convinced that she will suffer horribly were she to be told she has cancer. They confirmed my sense that in Greek culture, "cancer equals death"—something that in this case is in all likelihood true.

At this time the family was willing to sign any document we like assuming all responsibility for the decision to conceal the truth from Mrs. A. "Do us this one favor" was a plea that punctuated the discussion.

Discussion with the family was long and meandering. The usual position of the health care team was explained in some detail:

- Patients in our institution are generally told their diagnosis; we are accustomed to telling patients that they have cancer, and know how to handle the varied normal patient reactions to this bad news; patients do not (generally) kill themselves immediately upon being told or die a voodoo death, despite the family's fears and cultural beliefs about patient reaction to this diagnosis.
- Patients have a right to this information and may have the need to attend to any number of tasks pending death: to say goodbye, to make arrangements, to complete unfinished business.
- As her illness progresses, decisions will likely need to be made about further treatment: for example, as infections or blockages develop. Already, one of Mrs. A's kidneys is blocked and her urine is backing up. If the mass obstructs her other kidney, should a catheter be placed directly into the kidney or not? These decisions of treatment management for dying patients are dreadful and should if possible be made by the patient, in awareness of her choices and prospects.

In addition, Mrs. A is very likely already suspicious that she is gravely ill, and we have no means of dealing with her fears without the ability to speak to her openly. Finally, the fears that they expressed about the manner of informing her—"How can we tell our mother, 'You have cancer, it will kill you in weeks'?"—are groundless: She must be told that she is very ill, but we would never advise telling her she has a period of x weeks to live—a statement that is never wise, nor medically sound—nor will we try to remove her hope.

Despite all the explanations we provided to Mrs. A's family of the many reasons why it might be best to speak with her of her illness, they continued to resist. Mrs. A, the son insisted, would want all the decisions that arise to be made by the doctors, whom they all trust, and by the family itself.

If their assessment of Mrs. A is so, I pointed out, we have no problem. Dr. H agrees with me that while Mrs. A has a *right* to know, she does not have a *duty* to know. We would not force this information upon her—indeed, we cannot: Patients who don't want to know will sometimes deny ever having been told, however forthrightly they have been told of their condition. So Mrs. A will be offered this information, not have it thrust upon her; if they are right about what she wants and her personality, she will not ask questions about her condition.

Mrs. A was awake and reasonably alert, although not altogether free of discomfort (nausea). The doctor told her that she had an infection that was now under control, but that she remains very ill, as she herself can tell from her weakness. Does she have any questions she wants to ask; does she want to talk? She did not. We repeated that she remains very ill and asked if she understands that—she did.

Some patients, I explained to her, want to know all about their disease—its name, prognosis, treatment choices, famous people who have had the disease, etc.—while others do not want to know so much, and some want to leave all of the decisions in the hands of their family and doctors. What would she like? What kind of a patient is she? She whispered to her daughter that she wanted to leave it alone for now.

That seemed to be her final word. We repeated to her that treatment choices will need to be made shortly. She was told that we will respect her desire, but that if she changes her mind we can talk at any time; and that in any event, she must understand that we will stay by her and see to her comfort in all possible ways. She signified that she understood and said we should deal with her children. Both Dr. H and I understood her statement as explicitly authorizing her children to speak for her with respect to treatment decisions.

The family had earlier concocted a deal with Dr. H's predecessor; perhaps that physician had shared their view that Mrs. A should not be told the truth. It is predictable within our hospital system that such agreements will break down, either because the patient will need to be consulted during emergent circumstances, or because care of the patient will be transferred to another physician; eventual conflict is likely, if not inevitable. As is usual in conflict, the person wishing to change the status quo—in this case, Dr. H—requested the consultation. But in the midst of conflict, he was still bound together with the family in a common concern for the good of Mrs. A, and that was the topic of the ethics consultation.

The Consultation Process:
Some Differences Between the Models

Conflict and the Task of Consultations

In a regime of duty, in fact, conflict is attenuated; were there to exist a shared understanding of duty, indeed, conflict would be—in principle!—obviated altogether. A remarkable talmudic passage expresses this spirit. "Let he who comes from a court that has taken from him his cloak sing his song and go his way!"[9]—"sing his song" at his relief that he is no longer in possession of property that does not belong to him.

In a regime of rights, every conflict is a zero-sum game: For every winner, there must be a loser. Each rights claimant is making a personal assertion of power; each comes before the court saying, "I should have my way." Within a shared regime of duty, on the other hand, even civil conflict is framed in court as an honest inquiry, raised by two persons, over what the law requires.

This model, incidentally, fits well the reaction of Dr. H. He believed that it was his right to inform Mrs. A. (It is possible that in seeking the consultation this American-trained physician wished to confirm that Canada assigns rights in the same way that he had learned.) The result of the consultation confounded his expectations. But just as he recognized that Mrs. A has no duty to be informed of her cancer, he acknowledged that he himself had no duty to inform her of that fact. The surprising outcome of the consultation left him feeling reassured he had done his duty, and he too went his way "singing his song."

The model of duty thus helps to set the question, in ways that sometimes surprise the protagonists. What, after all, is a consultation about? What is "the question"? Within a model of rights, the question is inevitably narrowly construed as social ethics, hence, as the resolution of a defined conflict. The terms of discussion are set by the claims of those in conflict, and so innovative solutions tend to be ruled out of order.

In the second model, of expert consultancy, the terms of discussion are only somewhat broader. When that model privileges the moral perspective of one actor, usually the physician, the consultation can range over choices open to that person, whether previously considered or not; when the model admits other persons, their potential for action may be considered. Yet even then "the question" is: What shall the consultee, or consultees, *do*?

For the model of duty, by contrast, the first question is: What is to *be done*? and usually, in the clinical context: What is to be done for this patient? (The procedural question for the model of duty will be introduced in the following sections.) The model of duty thus broadens its focus, and its consultations tend to deal with an ongoing treatment plan rather than simply with an isolated issue or conflict. This seems to me useful, even if the precipitating cause of a consultation is a perceived conflict, for ethical conflicts have both a history and an aftermath, one of which needs to be acknowledged, the other managed.

Who Belongs in a Consultation?

A court, dealing with an isolated dispute, focuses its attention upon the narrowest possible question. The context of a clinical ethical consultation is less like a trial, whose litigants may afterward proceed their separate ways, and more like a conflict between neighbors. In the clinical context as in the neighborhood, the overt focus of conflict may be deceptive, with a long-standing undisclosed history of friction and mistrust that built up over time to the current *casus belli*. In both settings, too, once the current conflict is resolved the protagonists will need to find some way to continue to live with one another.

The number and identity of those who will be involved in a consultation are determined by the model adopted. By accepted principles of procedural justice, the model of rights will require the participation of the parties claiming rights in this matter, as well as input (although not necessarily participation) from those who can shed light upon it. As a model, expert consultancy is more flexible, although it will always necessarily begin (and, in practice, commonly conclude) with just the single person requesting the consultation. (Outside of the consultation per se, and adjunctive to it, the ethics consultant may of course be speaking with many others.)

The model of duty may of necessity entail broader participation. In this case of truth-telling in cancer, the discussion, begun with Dr. H, had to take place with the family members of the patient as well. But in its conclusion it may need to encompass many others, particularly nurses, other physicians, and other caregivers. The reason is that all of these share duties of caring for Mrs. A, and the object of the consultation—her right and proper care—requires coordination and cooperation between all of these.

This is a difference in kind, as well as in number. The consultation grounded in duty may be requested by different kinds of persons, for different reasons, than the other models could accommodate. The most striking example of this difference occurs when the patient is the person requesting the consultation.

ETHICS CONSULTATION: STOPPING DIALYSIS

I met with Mrs. L, at her request, following a suggestion to her by one of her nurses. Mrs. L, a woman in her seventies, is a veteran of the renal unit; she has been on dialysis for twenty years or more. She has developed a complication of long-term dialysis, amyloidosis, that causes her excruciating pain in her hands and feet. The question she wanted to discuss with me was simple and poignant: As a loving spouse and parent, when is enough enough? Many different efforts toward managing and controlling her pain have been tried, and all have failed sooner or later. Were she alone in the world, Mrs. L said, she would have stopped dialysis long ago, so she might die and be free of this constant torment. But her husband loves her and, she thinks, will fall apart without her companionship; and her children, although not similarly dependent upon her, will miss her terribly. Quite simply, she wanted to speak with someone about her obligations in this situation.

Biographies: Individuals Within Consultations

In general, it seems to me, a consultation grounded in an ethics of duty forces us to attend to the particularities of the persons involved. It is impossible to understand the problem posed in our case of Dr. G's patient who wanted to be allowed to die without knowing something of the biography of the protagonists: Dr. G's twenty-year professional relationship with Mrs. T, which had grown past mutual admiration and through to friendship. Dr. G's need to try one final ploy (a discussion of her wishes regarding resuscitation) before acceding to her wishes, and Mrs. T's forbearance with her doctor's ambivalence, only makes sense within an understanding of this relationship. The same may be said of the second case, in which her family wished to withhold from Mrs. A the fact that she had an advanced cancer. This family's cultural background was the essence of this discussion. A common theme in Greek families is concealment from and lying to those closest to you, from loving motives; as one family therapist experienced with that ethnic community writes, "Greek Americans do not believe that the truth shall make you free, and the therapist should not attempt to impose the love of truth upon them."[10] For his part, the specifics of Dr. H's professional moral commitments and ethical training were not irrelevant to his conflict with the family. Finally, the very fact of Mrs. L's question testified to her unusual family bonds and sense of responsibility.

What do I mean when I say that we "cannot make sense" of these issues without considering the biographies of those involved, and is this in any way distinctive of the model of duty, as opposed to those of rights and expert consultation? After all, any ethical approach will need to take account of the manner in which an ethical issue has arisen and the kinds of discussion to which protagonists are most likely to respond. For that matter, even if the theory of ethical consultation did not require such consideration, ordinary human sensitivity on the part of the consultant would supply it.

In the case of the model of duty, however, another dimension is added, for the biographies of the participants shape the very moral question posed. The duties incumbent upon Dr. G, Mrs. L, and all of the others are functions of their history, including—but extending beyond—their commitments, undertakings, and relationships. We need to know things about these people to understand the moral dilemmas they face: not, as in the model of rights, the basis upon which they make their assertions; not, as in the expert consultancy model, how they themselves understand their dilemmas; but rather, the nature, force, and outlines of the obligations themselves. Dr. G's obligations are not those of just any physician, and the satisfaction of his particular obligation to this specific patient will require him to take unusual steps.

Judaism and Consultations: Morality Within Relationships

Models and the Moral Persona

Let us approach this point from another angle. Both of the other models take persons as they choose (or chose) to present themselves. If the ethicist is an expert counselor to another, the terms are set by the client of the consultation. That client's persona is self-willed, and the history of the consultation is set by the client as well. (It was for that reason that Simpson, discussed earlier, cannot speak with patients or family members without his physician-client's consent.)

The model of rights poses a larger, and more interesting, problem. Its presence in ethics consultation is the merest epiphenomenon of an approach that underlies the major portion of our legal and political institutions. The subject of this model is an etiolated person, a possessor of bare rights, and this attenuated personum is self-willed in two ways. At the stage of the ethics consultation and thereafter, actors in this drama choose or decline to exercise their rights. Setting the stage for the consultation, moreover, the rights model understands persons as acquiring or losing rights on the basis of their free and uninhibited choices; the only kind of "duty" recognized within this model is that established by a freely chosen undertaking, upon the model of promising. This process extends back into the mythic past, to a point at which the very social rules establishing the structure of the rights model were themselves determined by choices of self-presentation, a decision to take certain acts as normatively binding. I cannot improve upon Robert Cover's exposition:

> The story behind the term "rights" is the story of social contract. The myth postulates free and independent if highly vulnerable beings who voluntarily trade a portion of their autonomy for a measure of collective security. The myth makes the collective arrangement the product of individual choice and thus secondary to the individual. "Rights" are the fundamental category because it is the normative category which most nearly approximates that which is the source of the legitimacy of everything else. Rights are traded for collective security.[11]

Morality Beyond Personal Choice: Judaism and Heteronomy

Not so—or, not simply so—for the model of duty. A duty can be acquired by voluntary choice, but its moral force is not exhausted by that choice. Dr. H chose to be a doctor, but need not have been aware of all the moral baggage that will come with that choice. In a model of rights he has a comeback—"I never consented!"—unavailable in a model of duties, which allows for moral consequences of living in certain ways, whether or not those lives are self-chosen, self-created, self-represented. As your life is shaped by forces, only some of which are subject to your influence, so is your moral life shaped. Cover writes of Judaism, as a paradigmatic system of duty,

The basic myth of Judaism is obligation or *mitzva*. It, too, is intrinsically bound up in a myth—the myth of Sinai. Just as the myth of social contract is essentially a myth of autonomy, so the myth of Sinai is essentially a myth of heteronomy. Sinai is a collective—indeed, a corporate—experience. The experience at Sinai is not chosen.[12]

(See the final portion of Section 2 for more on the choice at Sinai.)

Relationships can frame duties within this model; and it is true that the formation of relationships may be acts of self-will and even self-creation. Through certain acts, I had chosen, for example, to be a father, a choice that helped to set my world, including its moral parameters and my manner of living within it—to a degree, my being and identity. Other relationships also implicate duty, however, with no element of choice: I exist within the physical and moral worlds as a son, as a brother.

Duty Within Jewish Sources: Inescapably Relational

More remarkably, perhaps, the model of duty may force relationships where none had existed naturally, or by prior free choice. Certainly this is true within Judaism. The distinction between social and ritual duties is known within Judaism as the division of commandments into those *bein adam l'chaveiro* and those *bein adam lamakom,* literally translated, "between a man and his friend" and "between a man and the Omnipresent." It seems to an outsider that this first class of commandments deals with social duties, interpersonal behavior, but it is not understood that way in Jewish sources. Neutral phrases— "social" duties, "interpersonal" commandments, obligations to the "other"—are absent; instead, we hear of commandments regulating your behavior toward your *friend.* Human interactions are only understood as occurring between related persons. And more: The relations between persons are compelled, are Divinely ordained. And yet more: These persons in relationship are never *called* "persons." They exist within relationship and are named as such.

This tradition has its origins in the Bible. In introducing commandments, the neutral term *ezrach* (roughly corresponding to "citizen") is only used with reference to ritual commandments (such as celebrating the Festival of Booths). The term *ezrach* indeed seems to function as a placeholder for "person" to insist upon the equality of all, Jew and "stranger" alike, in ritual conditions that would otherwise establish inequality. (Compare, for example, the injunctions regarding the holidays of Sukkot and Yom Kippur, and the Temple service.)[13]

By contrast, no neutral terms are used to describe the protagonists of social duties. Instead, a vocabulary of relationship is imposed. Your duty to another is always described as your duty to your *ach,* your *'amit,* your *rei'a;* roughly translated, your brother, your friend, your neighbor.[14] Charity is not given to a "poor person" but rather to your *brother* who has become impoverished;[15] honest financial dealings occur between *friends;*[16] you are commanded not to oppress or steal from your *neighbor.*[17] The prohibition upon assault is not one imposed upon persons, citizens. Instead, the reader of the Bible is told that it is violated when "one man hit his *rei'a,*" his neighbor.[18]

We have a choice in how we shall understand this vocabulary. It may be that the reader is being told to act "as if" he or she were in relationship, as if the other were indeed your brother, friend, neighbor. That presumes that relationships must be self-created and that such self-created acts are the paradigm cases by analogy to which other forms of duty must be understood.[19] There is, however, another choice: These relationships do indeed exist, although not by your own choice; the Covenant has imposed them upon you. In one way, it matters little which understanding we adopt. Either way, the nature of obligations to the other is determined by one's life, not simply by one's own choices, by a rich persona existing within and defined by that person's life and much of its surroundings.

The Job of the Ethicist in the Jewish Model of Duty and Talmudic Formalism

In two ways, the role assigned the ethicist by the model of duty is distinctive: first, because the adjudication of duties is different from other normative tasks (notably, the parsing of rights); second, because the ethicist conducting a consultation is no less the object of duties than those others with whom he consults.

Within our society, an ethics consultation based upon rights relies, in a way, upon the courtroom looming in the background. The resolution of a consultation should mirror the conclusion a court would have reached; should the unsatisfied participants seek legal closure, the consult's conclusion should prefigure the decision the court does reach. But the judicial system will, potentially, not only validate these consultations but also enforce them. This is why successful consultations based upon the model of rights must have a winner and a loser. Their results must be isomorphic with comparable court cases.

In this respect, of course, duties are very different. The only powers an ethicist has within this model are those of clarification and persuasion. One writer sees this as key to the development of a duty-oriented Jewish jurisprudence. In the post-Exilic period Jewish courts had no instruments of physical coercion available to them, and for that reason the duty focus of Jewish law was crucial: "There the judge was not an umpire between adversaries; rather he was best qualified to tell the parties what behavior the Law prescribed for them, so as to prevent the erring party from committing a sin."[20]

As a statement regarding the jurisprudence of duties per se, this seems to me clearly mistaken: There is no barrier to the enforcement of duties, any more than to the enforcement of rights. But as regards the model of duties for ethics consultation, I think this exposition is right. The motivation with which a person agrees to such a consultation, the expectations he or she has, and the spirit within which the consultation is held are all influenced by this factor. Which is to say: Such a consultation is of no use to one determined to be proven right. Contrariwise, of course, the other models are of no use to one perplexed as to the right thing to do under the circumstances.

As a concomitant, Justice Moshe Silberg (of the Israeli Supreme Court) has claimed that the spirit of a jurisprudence of duty requires much more specific rules than does one grounded in rights. To borrow Justice Oliver Wendell Holmes's famous phrase, a law based upon rights satisfies the needs of "the bad man," the person who wants to know how he can maximally exercise his power without running afoul of the law.[21] By contrast, the scrupulous person is the proper object of a jurisprudence of duties, one who is focused upon the moral satisfaction of duties and obligations; and this person seeks rules precise enough that no court decision to ascertain whether a given deed is permitted will be needed.

This spirit, in Silberg's view, underlies talmudic formalism, the tendency of the Jewish jurisprudence of duty to track down every contingency and trace its moral ramifications. He illustrates this with a famous talmudic passage[22] dealing with the laws of found property. The rabbis ponder the case of a dove found in the vicinity of a dovecote; does it belong to the finder or to the owner of the dovecote, on the presumption that it is one of the latter's birds that had flown away? The Talmud sets a formal limit of fifty cubits rather than setting, as might have been done by a common-law court employing a jurisprudence of rights, a standard of "a reasonable distance," said standard to be applied by a court in considering all the facts of the case. That standard would serve well the needs of a "bad man," but it does no good to the scrupulous person; for, were the common-law "standard" approach to be adopted,

> What is he [the pigeon's finder] to do in order to decide whether he is obliged to return the young pigeon or not? It might be answered that he does not have to do anything; he may just wait until the other party sues him, and then the matter will be fully clarified through the procedure described above. True, he may do so, but only if his sole concern is that the other person might sue him, and that he will end up having to return what he found and pay the cost of the trial in addition. This is the ordinary problem, confronting the ordinary citizen, in every ordinary state. But what if this is not the case, if the question is from the outset not one of *law* but one of *conscience,* if this particular finder wishes to maintain peace with himself and to know whether he is under the duty of fulfilling the religious-moral precept of returning a lost object? . . . It is not the right of a person to something which is the determining and determined thing, but the duty of the person under obligation—how and under what conditions he has to fulfill his religious or moral duty toward another.

Therefore the measures stated in the law must be fixed and determinate, weighed and precisely evaluated, measures which every ordinary person will be able to use without the necessity of approaching the judge for interpretation.[23]

In his final statement, Justice Silberg seems to have overstepped the mark. The proliferation of rules and the detailed consideration of cases provided in Jewish texts does not seem to have obviated the need for rabbinic guidance and interpretation: To the contrary, it often seems to have fostered that need, in a positive feedback loop. Rules, however specific, are not self-interpreting. But Silberg's premise is valid: One oriented toward duty seeks more, rather than less, moral guidance, whether provided through a more specific rule, through easier access to assistance in interpreting the rule, or otherwise. In this way, the ethicist working with a model of duty plays a distinctive role, as regards both goals and moral raw materials. The following sections are intended in part to draw out some of the implications of this distinctness.

The Moral Stance of the Consulting Ethicist

As a last point of difference between the models, consider the moral stance attached to clinical ethicists themselves. The following case challenged my own moral stance in a number of ways.

ETHICS CONSULTATION: FEEDING IN STROKE—
ASK HER NO QUESTIONS

A telephone call from Nurse A triggered this consultation. She had spoken to me before the New Year of the patient and of associated ethical issues, but no discussion was held at that time. She felt the new issues were more serious and needed attention. The patient, Mrs. C, had not had a feeding tube for several previous days, and there was no intention of reinserting it; indeed, other members of the health team have made Nurse A feel like she is making too much of a fuss about this case. She provided at that time some further details, which I will fold into the following discussion. On the basis of what she told me, I assured her this was a serious case that should have a discussion.

Contrary to my policy up to that point, I took the initiative and called Dr. F to ask him to come in for a discussion about the care of Mrs. C and arranged for the others to come to the meeting as well. Mrs. C is a ninety-one-year-old woman who had been quite functional (although she needed help with activities of daily living) and had been a resident of a skilled nursing facility for the previous seventeen years. She was transferred to our hospital for a hip repair. However, before the surgery could be performed, she suffered a serious stroke that has left her hemiplegic [partially paralyzed] and aphasic [unable to speak], as well as without a gag reflex [unable to avoid breathing in food or drink when she swallows]. She was reassigned to long-term care in January. The prognosis, given the extent of her stroke, is poor, and she is not expected to regain function sufficient for discharge. She appears to be comfortable and has a private sitter with her at all times. There has been a problem in keeping her feeding tube in; she has pulled it out three times, with the usual accompanying delays in reinsertion. For some reason that was not explained, she was not considered a candidate for gastrostomy [surgical insertion of a feeding tube into her stomach]. She also suffers from Parkinson's disease, but she has no other active disease process under way and could live for a prolonged period with adequate care and nutrition. The nurses believe she is alert, but she cannot speak. Nurse A, at my request, had checked before the meeting whether she was consistently responsive to yes/no questions, and Nurse A claims she was: She touches her chin or nods to signify yes, touches her wrist or shakes her head for no.

The only family remaining to Mrs. C are two nieces and a nephew, all in Montreal; further relatives live elsewhere. The family has said that Mrs. C should be kept comfortable, but not have her life artificially prolonged. At one point they told the staff that they had asked her if she wants to die, and she said that she did. The day before I was called one niece sent in a letter stating that it was the unanimous family wish that she not have the feeding tube reinserted.

At the outset of our discussion, Nurse A emphasized that she is very concerned. She felt that the family was not making a decision that was in Mrs. C's interests; she is in all events unhappy at the thought of a patient of hers starving to death, an approach she considers to be cruel and an affront to her professional moral identity. She thought it possible that the family has a conflict of interest regarding this very wealthy aunt. Her feelings were not totally without ambivalence, though, based upon the view others expressed to her that this was no real issue. The social worker felt the family members were involved, close, and caring, but in response to Nurse A's point about conflict of interest, thought some conflict was possible.

Dr. F thought the letter from the family was the end of the story legally, though he expressed some ethical discomfort with the outcome. One niece said that she had power of attorney and was acting on that basis. I disagreed that the letter settled anything. Power of attorney was not equivalent to a mandate granting medical decision-making authority, which probably had not been effected. It was true that nonetheless under our law these family members probably qualified as proxy decision makers; however, they are only permitted to consent to or refuse treatment taking into account the patient's interest and expressed wishes. It was certainly arguable that not feeding her was contrary to her best interest; if we felt so, we have an obligation to seek authority from the public curator's office for treatment and feeding. In addition, Nurse A disclosed that last Friday the nephew revealed to her that he was only going along with the wishes of the nieces; as for him, he felt that Mrs. C's life was worthwhile, in at least a spiritual sense. However, he would not stand in their way. Thus, we do not know whether the family is unanimous or in which fashion unanimity was achieved.

Dr. Y was more comfortable substantively with respecting the family wishes. She felt that Nurse A exaggerated the discomfort associated with failing to provide nutrition, and that this discomfort needs in any case to be considered in relation to that caused by the feeding tube. Mrs. C would not live long or well in any event; looking at the chart, she noted that Mrs. C appears to have had several previous small strokes, accumulating damage.

As an initial resolution, I suggested that we see if Mrs. C can express her own preference. We all felt it was inappropriate to ask her if she wants to die. She could, however, be shown the feeding tube; we could explain to her that this is the only way we have to feed her, and she could be asked if she wants us to put it back in. Dr. Y was dubious as to whether she would understand the question or give a knowing response, but given Nurse A's examination prior to the meeting, it nonetheless seemed a possibility, however remote. Those at the bedside would have to make a judgment call as to whether the patient seems alert and knowingly responsive; whether, that is, her behavior is a meaningful response to the questions posed. Nurse A was somewhat hesitant about how to react in the event of a negative response, but all agreed after a little discussion that a genuine decision from Mrs. C in either direction must be respected.

Left in some limbo was the question of what would be done if she didn't respond; it seemed to me, on reflection and after talking with the hospital's director of professional services, that we would need to have a family meeting to clarify the implication of the decision and to ascertain their current and true feelings.

I spoke to Nurse A later that afternoon. She described the scene at the bedside: A whole bevy of personnel were around to witness the event. Mrs. C unambiguously signified that she wanted the feeding tube put back in, and Dr. F wrote a note to that effect in the chart.

On Friday I received another phone call from Nurse A. For some reason she did not know, Dr. F had not written the order for feeding on Tuesday. The family members had been told of this discussion with Mrs. C, though, and were very much opposed to the resolution. They did not believe that she in fact understood and meaningfully responded to the question about feeding, nor that she wishes to live. They claimed that, as an old French Québécois family (de vieille souche) in a French province, this Jewish hospital has no right to impose its values upon them. They demanded that feeding not be reinstated until a discussion with Mrs. C would be held at which they would be present, as well as their family doctor. This could not take place before the following Wednesday. The family was indeed well-connected. They had arranged for a senior bureaucrat of the Ministry of Health to call Dr. F and caution him regarding this case. Apparently, Dr. F had been acceding to their demands in not yet reinstating the tube. The nurse wanted to know my reaction to this.

I asked Nurse A if she could review the chart to see if Mrs. C seemed to be at risk at this time. Her urea was down a little but her studies otherwise looked about right. I told Nurse A that it may be fine for the family to observe a repeat of the interchange about feeding, but that I was concerned that they not intimidate Mrs. C by their presence. My suggestion was that the interchange be reenacted with the family present in the doorway where they might see and hear what is going on but where Mrs. C would not see them. However, I was concerned about the delay all this involves. She had already been off feeding by this time for some eight days, and if feeding would not begin until after this meeting, it would be two weeks. I did not know if this was dangerous, and, more to the point, did not know if there was anything I could do about it. I promised the nurse I would make some calls, but told her I was not sure what, if anything, might come of this.

I immediately called Dr. Y to tell her of developments and ask her about the situation. She felt that each day off feeding at this point was a substantial risk and thought now that the resolution should be to reinstate feeding until the family meeting or until Mrs. C pulled out the tube again. I then camped out at the office of the director of professional services, who was at that time between meetings. I caught him for a few minutes, and informed him of what has transpired. He understood the sense of urgency I had about this. He agreed to try to contact Dr. F. He could not instruct him to feed—as the patient's responsible physician, Dr. F has authority over medical orders—but he could make sure Dr. F had a good reason if he fails to do so. We also talked about our shared sense that my action in this case may be out of line with my role as a clinical ethicist and agreed to discuss that on some future occasion. The director of professional services called me at home late in the afternoon to tell me he had reached Dr. F, who agreed to insert a tube that day.

On the following Wednesday a meeting was held with Dr. F, the family, their doctor, Nurse A, and the hospital's patient representative. I heard about the meeting afterward from the director of professional services and from the patient representative. The family were very huffy and oppositional, and their doctor even more so. He went on at some length about how the patient has the right to die and the hospital is not justified in interfering. Dr. F's conduct was described as a model of diplomacy in handling them and explaining the basis on which he had acted. A discussion was then held around the bedside of Mrs. C. She was described as having some difficulty knowing whom she is supposed to please, and in that sense, the patient representative thought my suggestion that they observe but not be around was borne out. Notwithstanding, Mrs. C expressed a clear desire to live and to be fed, in response to yes/no questions. The scene was described as "like out of some movie." Those present were touched, misty-eyed, and the family seemed now to have a real sense that there is a person there with present desires for feeding and treatment. The meeting ended amicably, although nobody apologized for their oppositional stance. I heard on February 26 that Mrs. C is still comfortable and doing as well as might be expected.

Mrs. C was subsequently transferred back to a convalescent home. I last saw Nurse A some two and a half years following this case consultation, and at that time the patient was still residing within that home.

I have discussed elsewhere the remarkable reluctance of those writing on clinical ethics to state the circumstances that would require an ethicist to act upon the dictates of his or her own conscience.[24] Was I acting rightly as an ethicist in this case? This is an uncannily difficult problem for one employing the expert consultation model, as is revealed in this comment by Edmund Howe, discussing

> whether the ethics consultant should assert a definitive position and insist that others adopt his position or remain more neutral, primarily clarifying alternatives. The former approach is more likely to protect an individual patient's immediate interests in the short run, but it may alienate the physician and deprive the ethics consultant of opportunities to help a greater number of patients in the long run.[25]

The question seems much simpler for those following a model of rights; the ethicist should be concerned to see that possessors of rights are vindicated. As Robertson writes, "At some point, the duty to report wrongdoing may even cause the ethicist to risk his or her job."[26]

For either model, however, it is arguable that action on behalf of a patient's welfare or even rights goes beyond the ethicist's job description. Even within the rights model, the ethicist clarifies and explores patient's rights; it is as a person, not as an ethicist, that he or she might be obliged to secure rights.

Reflecting upon this case, I have concluded that even this tenuous distinction is not available for the model of duty. An ethicist within that understanding—my understanding—may discover his own commitments and sense of moral duty to be engaged, just as is true for other participants.

These, then, are some of the structural differences between an ethical approach grounded in rights and one based upon duties. But as has been said above, that which is most distinctive about an ethics of duty, such as Judaism, is the substantive way in which it formulates those duties. In the following sections, I turn to that task.

Endnotes

1. A distinction is drawn by some between obligations, which are self-assumed moral responsibilities (as in promises or contracts), and duties, which are moral responsibilities consequent upon the social role one occupies (as in professional or familial responsibilities). I will ignore this distinction in what follows.*

2. Compare with Robert M. Veatch, "The Ethics of Institutional Ethics Committees," in *Institutional Ethics Committees and Health Care Decision Making*, eds. Ronald Cranford and Edward Doudera (Ann Arbor, MI: Health Administration Press, 1984): 35–50 at 42.*

3. Terrence Ackermann, "Moral Problems, Moral Inquiry, and Consultation in Clinical Ethics," in *Clinical Ethics: Theory and Practice*, eds. Barry Hoffmaster, Benjamin Freedman, and Gwen Fraser (Clifton, NJ: Humana Press, 1989): 155–157.

4. James F. Drane, "Hiring a Hospital Ethicist," in *Ethics Consultation in Health Care*, eds. John C. Fletcher, Norman Quist, and Albert R. Jonsen (Ann Arbor, MI: Health Administration Press, 1989): 117–134.

5. Kenneth Simpson, "The Development of a Clinical Ethics Consultation Service in a Community Hospital," *Journal of Clinical Ethics* 3, no. 2 (1992): 124–130.

6. E. Pellegrino, M. Siegler, and P. Singer, *Journal of Clinical Ethics* 2, no. 1 (1991): 6–7.

7. See Courtney S. Campbell and B. Andrew Lustig, eds., *Duties to Others* (Dordrecht, The Netherlands: Kluwer Academic Publishers, 1994).*

8. See Benjamin Freedman, "Offering Truth: One Ethical Approach to the Uninformed Cancer Patient," *Archives of Internal Medicine* 135 (1993): 572.*

9. TB *Sanhedrin* 7a.

10. E. P. Welts, "The Greek Family," in *Ethnicity and Family Therapy*, eds. M. M. McGoldrick, J. K. Pearce, and J. Giordano (New York: Guilford Press, 1982): 269–288.

11. Robert Cover, "Obligation: A Jewish Jurisprudence of the Social Order," *Journal of Law and Religion* 5 (1988): 65–74, at 66.

12. Cover (1988).*

13. Sukkot: Lev. 23.42; Yom Kippur: Lev. 16.29; Temple service: Num. 15.29.

14. Compare with commentary on Lev. 19.18 in R Samson Raphael Hirsch, *Commentary on the Torah*, trans. Isaac Levy (Gateshead, England: Judaica Press, 1973).*

15. Lev. 25.35; Deut. 15.7.

16. Lev. 5.20.

17. Ex. 19.13.

18. Ex. 21.18.

19. But self-created acts may themselves be compulsory, as can be found in exploring the paradox of the imposed consent within Judaism. See TB *Avoda Zara* 2b.*

20. Translator's introduction, Moshe Silberg, "Law and Morals in Jewish Jurisprudence," *Harvard Law Review* 75 (1961): 306–331 at 307.

21. Oliver Wendell Holmes, Jr., *The Common Law* (London: Macmillan, 1882).

22. TB *Bava Batra* 23b.

23. Silberg (1961): 325–327.

24. Benjamin Freedman, "From Avocation to Vocation: Working Conditions for Clinical Bioethicists," in *The Health Care Ethics Consultant*, ed. Françoise Baylis (Totowa, NJ: Humana Press, 1994): 109–132.

25. Edmund G. Howe, "When Physicians Impose Values on Patients: An Ethics Consultant's Responsibilities," in *Ethics Consultation in Health Care*, eds. John C. Fletcher, Norman Quist, and Albert R. Jonsen (Ann Arbor, MI: Health Administration Press, 1989): 137–148 at 137.

26. John A. Robertson, "Clinical Medical Ethics and the Law: The Rights and Duties of Ethics Consultants," in *Ethics Consultation in Health Care*, eds. John C. Fletcher, Norman Quist, and Albert R. Jonsen (Ann Arbor, MI: Health Administration Press, 1989): 149–172 at 168.

FAMILY

the role of the family in medical decision making for incompetent persons

Introduction

In the Prologue, I began this exploration of a Jewish approach to bioethics by considering the nature of the clinical ethics consultation. I argued that a model of duty provides a more useful description of that peculiar interaction than alternative understandings can: An ethical consultation is best understood as an effort on the part of those caring for a patient to discover what their obligations to the patient require and how these obligations can best be satisfied. That discussion revolved around what is admittedly a fringe phenomenon—the formal ethics consultation—and failed to explore the nature of the claims of duty with which it deals. This section will take one further step toward understanding how specific duties are central to bioethical issues.

Decision Making for Competent and Incompetent Patients

If we had to choose the single most common and difficult ethical issue posed in the hospital, it would undoubtedly be the appropriate care of the incompetent patient. This is the reason why bioethics so often focuses upon the beginning and the end of life, in particular, on treatment issues concerning infants and the dying elderly patient.

Within our society, with its commitment to autonomy and its identification of ethics with social ethics, we rarely discern any ethical issue in complying with self-regarding treatment decisions by competent patients. Most seeming exceptions to that rule turn out, upon closer examination, to fall outside its scope. While many ethical issues arise from psychiatric patients' refusal of treatment, for example, this is largely because of uncertainty over their status as competent decision makers. Those who see ethical issues in complying with the wishes of patients who demand futile treatment usually feel these demands are not fully self-regarding, either because satisfying them will consume resources better spent for other purposes or because the health care provider satisfying these demands is thereby compelled to violate his or her canons of professional integrity. And again, the ethical controversy regarding compliance with patient requests for euthanasia or physician-assisted suicide is in large part grounded in doubts about either or both of the qualifications I stated earlier: Is the patient expressing a true and competent wish? Is the request self-regarding in its effect, or will its satisfaction impact others within society in undesirable ways?

As a general rule, then, competent patients making decisions on their own behalf are not a major source of bioethical interest. Whatever moral problems such decisions may raise are questions for patients to deal with on their own; rightly or wrongly, these personal questions need not be discussed by others.

When the patient is not competent to decide, however, the problem of treatment decisions is seen as public fare: Who should decide, and how, and on the basis of which moral principles, and with what safeguards? The context in which treatment decisions for incompetent patients arise conspires to make them peculiarly difficult. The category of "incompetent patient" encompasses the infant or young child, the adult in the throes of profound psychosis, the demented geriatric patient, the comatose victim of an accident or assault, the patient in the end stage of a terminal disease like cancer who is rendered incoherent by illness or medication, and others. These voiceless persons are among the most vulnerable members of society. Historically, they have been frequent victims of discriminatory neglect and abuse. Their voiceless condition is often the consequence of profound, systemic bodily malfunctioning. Therefore, the problems of treatment and medical management they raise are complex; their stay in hospital or under close medical supervision, prolonged; their prognosis, often poor; the therapy and palliative care they require, astronomically expensive. It is no coincidence that bioethics has been preoccupied with the ethical issues raised in the care of the incompetent.

The Role of Family Members

Here we will consider the role of family members in reaching treatment decisions on behalf of the incompetent patient. While the question remains the focus of much debate, there has nonetheless emerged an approach held by so many and so deeply as to amount to the standard view, the received wisdom. That view holds that the usual characteristics of families—their knowledge of and concern for the interests of their members—cause families to seek, and the law to ratify, a defeasible right for their participation in treatment decisions on behalf of incompetent members. This is by no means a simple claim. I want to consider, and to question, some of the several premises upon which it rests and to propose an alternative understanding of the role of families, one grounded in a Jewish understanding of family obligations.

As before, a case will help us focus our attention upon this problem. The one I present was chosen because of the meaning it held for me and the impact it had upon my views. It is not typical of the category in several ways; for example, it does not turn upon a life-and-death dilemma associated with the use of high-technology medicine. In its human and relevant moral aspects, however, it poses the same questions as any case dealing with the voiceless: Who should intervene, when, how, with what warrant, and on the basis of which principles?

ETHICS CONSULTATION: THE SAD TALE OF A PRODIGY

I had met Ms. M at a talk I gave to Jewish Family Service concerning ethical issues, at which time she raised a difficult case of hers and asked whether I would agree to meet with her and her client.

The discussion concerned an approach to Ben, Mr. C's son. Mr. C is ninety years old and lives in Montreal with his wife (not Ben's mother, who died when Ben was young). Mr. C's daughter, Mrs. L, lives in rural Quebec and appears to be in her late fifties. Ben himself is sixty years old and lives alone in Montreal.

Ben was a child prodigy in science and mathematics, and as a young man enjoyed international success and recognition. His father and sister disagree on whether there were early signs of his illness. Undisputed is that by the early 1970s he had persistent odd beliefs, which appear to have contributed to his divorce at that time. He proceeded upon a downhill course from that point, culminating in a frank psychotic break during a lecture tour in Europe in 1979, at which time the police picked him up, naked and suffering from exposure, in a city park. Mr. C was fortunate to procure the services of a psychiatrist who flew overseas to bring Ben back to Montreal. That psychiatrist treated Ben for a brief time at his hospital with oral medication. The daughter recalls that the diagnosis at that time included paraphrenia. It appears that the treating psychiatrist encouraged Mr. C to sign papers discharging Ben from the hospital on the understanding that Ben would continue his medication. Ben himself was very anxious to be released from the hospital. He was discharged, but it proved impossible to maintain Ben's compliance with medication.

Ben has been living on his own for many years now. He would frequently take the bus to visit his father; this is a bit awkward because Mr. C's wife is a fastidious woman who sounds uncomfortable about having Ben around, having to clean up after him, and so on. He has had no medical attention that anyone knows of since the above-noted hospitalization. Mr. C has not visited him in his apartment and believes Ben would not let him in because of shame at its unkempt state. Ben's landlord knows of his oddities and tolerates them. His rent has always been paid and he has been, broadly speaking, an acceptable tenant. Mrs. L, Ben's sister, has gone to see him from time to time without her father and speaks to him by phone.

Some two weeks ago, Ben did not appear at an appointed time at his father's home. Coming later, he told a rambling tale of satellites and bombs and his sister's dying but then not dying and . . . A variety of his several delusions were incorporated, in a way and with perhaps an undertone of violence, that alarmed Mr. C. Mr. C's wife told him that this nonsense was frightening her husband, and Ben thereupon left.

Mr. C met with Ms. M, apparently to inquire about how to get treatment for Ben, whom he feels has clearly been getting worse. Ms. M has met with Ben and has seen his apartment, which is in a horribly filthy and ill-kept state. Ben is thin but appears to be in reasonable health.

A long and often touching discussion ensued. Mr. C confirmed that he is both concerned about Ben's current state but perhaps even more about Ben's getting worse later at a time when Mr. C himself, given his current advanced age, would no longer be able to keep an eye out for him. Tearfully, he explained how he understands that Ben will not become what he once was. He simply hopes for enough improvement so he can speak sensibly with his son once again.

Pros and cons of treatment options for Ben were discussed. Ms. M's observation of Ben indicates that despite the degraded condition in which he lives, he is reasonably content. Mr. C explained how Ben is sometimes tranquil but at other times is tormented by contortions demanded of him by his delusions. It emerged clearly that seeking a court order for involuntary hospitalization would cause Ben much anguish. It was by no means clear that treatment could be offered to him even then (given in part his unknown medical condition), on what kind of prolonged basis, to what effect, and with what side effects. All present agreed that the harm-benefit ratio of this course of action now was not favorable. I discussed the various reasons for instituting any form of treatment—prolongation of life, restoring function, treating uncomfortable symptoms—and what these might imply in Ben's own case.

A resolution was reached for Mr. C to restore contact with Ben, together with a social worker to be assigned to the case, who would offer him some instruction and practice in avoiding speaking about and confrontation over the delusions. This will be important in providing a bridge between Mr. C (who has until this time been the primary caregiver) and whoever might play that role in the future. Efforts to persuade Ben to agree to see a physician will be made. Were Ben to agree to see a doctor and try treatment, it is possible that he could experience some relief from his symptoms.

I raised the question of Ben's finances. The welfare check of psychiatric patients is sometimes sent to the patient's psychiatrist, ensuring that the patient will not lose all contact with the doctor. Ms. M pointed out that this would require first the same court order and forced transfer to a facility for treatment, and so that idea was rejected. (At some later point, however, it was arranged that Ben's check would be sent to his social worker, Ms. M, an arrangement that served to much the same effect.) This status quo was recognized to be a measure that would need to be watched closely, and it was also recognized that involuntary treatment might have to be instituted at some point, for example, if Ben's condition becomes life-threatening to him.

In early October Mr. C came to see me again. His son had been evicted from his apartment in August and had refused to take an apartment across the street that was arranged. He refused to leave his apartment, the police were called, and he was hospitalized at our hospital for four days under a court order. He was not excessively agitated, and so his refusal of medication was not overridden. He had been released after four days. While hospitalized, he refused to see his father; he told him, "I will find a place to stay, and then I'll call you." On September 1 he showed up at his old apartment to collect his welfare check, but he has not resurfaced since then. He has not gone back for October, and welfare says he never sent back a card with current whereabouts. Mr. C was acutely anxious when he came to see me; he didn't know what to do.

I called the social worker while he was in my office; since Mr. C is very hard of hearing, I was able to speak freely. She confirmed that matters were basically as he described. While she herself is concerned, she didn't feel anything should be done at this time. She had contacted the patient's sister, who was confident that he would reappear unharmed; she thought he had probably traveled to Ottawa. She had not checked hospitals in Montreal or Ottawa to see if Ben had been admitted. I told her that in my gut I felt something should be done. She explained that Mr. C would have to go to the police himself to report his son as missing, and this would be very hard for him. (I didn't see it as any harder than what he's going through now.) We did agree that if he missed his November check concern would be much more appropriate, and there would be no question that action was needed, irrespective of the patient's sister's view.

I spoke some more with Mr. C, explaining the recommendation. He felt awful about his son's refusing to see him while hospitalized, thinking his son blamed him—wrongly—for the involuntary hospitalization. I reminded him that the son had at times tried to avoid having his father see him in distressing or humiliating circumstances, and this was probably the reason in this case as well. He left, I felt, somewhat reassured—whereas I felt badly thinking there is no basis for reassuring him now, while not knowing what else to do.

I saw Ms. M at a lecture the evening of October 21, and spoke again briefly. She agreed they had waited long enough, and it was time for Mr. C., accompanied by his geriatric social worker, to make a police report.

In the following years, I have seen Ms. M and have been visited by Mr. C a number of times. One kind of closure occurred just a few months before this writing: Mr. C, now well into his nineties, was admitted to hospital after suffering a major stroke, and Ms. M, who had successfully found and maintained contact with Ben, wanted to discuss whether she should inform him of this fact and try to persuade him to come to the hospital.

A Proper Family Role: The Standard View

Abstracting away some of the unusual circumstances of this case, the questions it poses are reasonably common. How aggressively should treatment options be pursued? at what expense to the patient, as measured primarily in pain and loss of dignity and freedom? to what purpose, and for how long? Questions of this same kind underlie such issues as whether to artificially ventilate a highly premature neonate with serious intraventricular hemorrhage who stops breathing, and whether to tube-feed a patient with advanced senile dementia of the Alzheimer's type (SDAT) who can no longer swallow by herself and who will need to be restrained to prevent her from pulling out her feeding tube.

In addition to these substantive issues, the case of Ben raises the same procedural questions as do other cases of treatment decisions for incompetent persons. The first of these procedural questions is: Who should decide? Ben's father, Mr. C, was assigned or allowed the role of surrogate medical decision maker by the social worker. This meant that the main "treatment" choices in this case—namely, when to mobilize the medico-legal resources available to arrange psychiatric and medical treatment for Ben—were left up to Mr. C's judgment.

A number of questions that could be posed at this point, both substantive and procedural, will not be addressed in the following discussion. I will not deal with the question of whether the decisions reached by Mr. C were substantively correct nor, for example, whether Ms. M's (and my own) acceptance of Mr. C as his son's surrogate decision maker was reasonable. Ben's sister, Mrs. L, could have claimed this privilege for herself (although she did not); other family members or significant others could have stepped forward.

The Basis for a Family Role

Rather, I want to concentrate upon this issue: On what basis may *any* family member be allowed to make medical decisions for an incompetent person? When we ask for the basis of a family's role, however, we may be asking two different things: the normative warrant for the family's role or the reasons underlying a family's role. The first question has its stock answer: Ultimately, within our society, any legal power, whatever its genesis, eventuates in claims of right; the role of the family is no different in this respect. Observe how the writer in the following passage, all unnoticed, passes from an assertion that the family has a *responsibility* to decide to the view that the family claims a *right* to decide:

> [M]edical determinations for incompetent patients should be within the family's sphere of *responsibility.* . . . The common

law doctrine of informed consent, more recently supplemented by the constitutional right of privacy, acknowledges the *rights* of patients or their surrogates to resolve health care questions.[1]

While this passage explains the nature of the role families will be assigned, it does not provide the reasons why families should have a role in decision making. The standard response to this latter question is perhaps best expressed by Buchanan and Brock, in their outstanding discussion of treatment decisions for incompetent persons:

> The chief reasons in support of the presumption that the family is to serve as surrogate decision-maker are both obvious and compelling. The family is generally both most knowledgeable about the incompetent individual's good and his or her previous values and preferences, and most concerned about the patient's good. Furthermore, especially in a society in which impersonal relationships have replaced most other forms of community, participation in the family as an intimate association is one important way in which individuals find or construct meaning in their lives. Since intimate relationships can only thrive under conditions of privacy, society should be reluctant to intrude in the family's decisions concerning its own members, unless others are adversely affected.[2]

Three separate rationales are provided here; restated, Buchanan and Brock claim that decisions about an incompetent member's medical treatment should be determined by members of his or her family because:

1. Families are an important social unit within our society, and their private decisions should in general be respected.[3]
2. Family members can be trusted, because they are concerned about the welfare of their members, to choose those treatments and medical decisions that will protect the best interests of the incompetent patient.[4]

3. The close and prolonged interaction that takes place within families results in family members being the best qualified to judge how the incompetent patient would have responded to the same medical choice had he or she been capable of responding.[5]

What Kind of Decisions Are Family Decisions?

Of these reasons, the first is conceptually the weakest. We can agree that family decisions should be respected, particularly at this historical juncture. The family unit is under great stress, and the support it can provide is arguably more needed now than ever. But the question was: Why should families be allowed to make these decisions? The answer given is: Because families should be left free to make family decisions. The response simply begs the question: Why are decisions about an incompetent person's medical care *family* decisions? Granted, some medical decisions take place in the privacy of the home, as when a parent decides to take an infant with a cough to the doctor for an examination. But the decisions with which we are concerned are different: They concern persons who are hospitalized, live in institutions, or at any event are under close and regular medical supervision.

It is true that there is no simple demarcation here. We cannot simply say, for example, that all decisions occurring and fulfilled at home are family decisions, and those outside are not. But in noticing the complexity of the distinction between those decisions families are empowered to make unilaterally regarding the lives of their members and those subject to outside surveillance, investigation, and control, we are forced to recognize the socially constructed nature of that distinction. In some societies, at some times, an adult child's choices of residence, spouse, and employment were all "family decisions," that is, subject to parental (paternal) control, similar to whether and how a minor child would be educated.

The ambit of family control is a matter that, in a changing society, is always up for rational discussion. Calls to maintain or to change the status quo must be judged on the basis of supporting reasons. (Indeed, even to say what *is* the status quo is difficult regarding some choices, as in the clinical context, that have never been faced before.) The reasons given may be good or bad, and "because it's always been done that way" is not on the positive side of that divide. But Buchanan and Brock didn't even say that. What they did say is that decisions about the treatment of an incompetent patient should be made by the family because they are family decisions. This doesn't even provide us with a bad reason for the proposition; by the canons of logic, it provides no reason at all.

"Best Interest" and "Substituted Judgment" as a Basis for Decisions

The second and third reasons are more effective. They derive from a dispute regarding the substantive principles that should govern medical decision making on behalf of an incompetent person. According to one view, the criterion should be the patient's best interest. The surrogate (whoever that might be) should choose the medical course of action most likely to maximally contribute to the patient's welfare. The alternative view (known opaquely in legal circles as the "doctrine of substituted judgment") has argued that the surrogate should reach that decision which the incompetent patient would have chosen had he or she been competent. Court decisions may be found favoring either of these views, as well as a variety of confusing efforts at their merger or reconciliation.

I have elsewhere discussed this issue, and have concluded by favoring a "best-interests" approach.[6] For our present procedural purposes, however, this substantive issue need not be settled, as Buchanan and Brock argue that the family is the unit best situated to apply either criterion. Family members are both concerned for the incompetent patient's best interests and knowledgeable regarding those factors (e.g., her values, beliefs, and preferences) that would have caused her (were she competent) to have decided in a certain way.

What Are the Limits of Family Authority? The Standard View

As mapmaking is not concluded until the boundaries have been inked in, we cannot claim to understand this standard view of the family's role without having described its limits. In other words:

Under which circumstances, according to the standard view, should a family no longer be permitted to make these decisions? When do their decisions need to be subject to review, and ultimate approval or veto, by outsiders (such as a hospital ethics committee, a government tribunal, or a judge)?

Buchanan and Brock describe a broad range of such exceptions, which they term "intervention principles." In their understanding, some cases intrinsically require outside review, whatever the decision reached by the family—for example, when the patient in question has been institutionalized for a lengthy period or when the choice faced has great and irreversible consequences, as when deciding about surgical sterilization of an incompetent person. Sometimes, outside intervention is needed because the specific decision reached by the family seems unreasonable—for example, those decisions that are contrary to a consensus of physicians involved in the case or that seem clearly contrary to the patient's interests and previous desires. In addition, any and all family members may lose their right to participate in decisions about a patient's treatment for any one of a number of reasons: because they themselves lack the capacity to understand and meaningfully weigh the medical choice in question (i.e., because they are themselves incompetent), because they have abused or neglected the patient or have failed to demonstrate any strong family attachment to the patient, or because the decision places them in a serious conflict of interest with the patient.[7]

The logical basis of these intervention principles is transparent. Families have been chosen to serve as decision makers for incompetent patients because they may be trusted to safeguard the welfare and values of their members. Whenever there is reason to question whether they can be trusted to fulfill these tasks, outside review and ratification are necessary.

Limits to Family Authority: The Legal Approach

Within the legal arena, both courts and legislatures have adopted similar principles. For example, the New York Supreme Court Appelate Division writes that the appointment of a stranger "is in the best interests of the incompetent where the record discloses dissension

in the family, the adverse interests of the relatives and the incompetent . . . or any other reason whereby a stranger would best serve the
interest of the incompetent."[8] The courts have paid particular attention to describing those circumstances under which a family is disqualified because of their conflict of interest.[9] They include cases where:

- Treatment decisions may be influenced by the potential financial impact upon the family which they entail.[10]
- The effect of treatment decisions upon the family's other
  children may unduly influence the family's judgment.[11]
- The family's judgment may be influenced by their hopes
  to speedily inherit the patient's property.[12]

Legislatures have similarly been alert to the need to disqualify
families under defined (but often very broad) circumstances. Even
those legislatures that have defined the order in which family members are to be approached for the task of decision making (commonly,
for example, the right is held in the first instance by husband or wife;
if none is available, by adult child; if none is available, by sibling,
etc.), have explicitly provided for these priorities to be disregarded if
an apprehension is present that the patient's best interests will not
thereby be served.[13] The concern persists; as one commentator on a
recent New York State legislative proposal writes, "[T]he review apparatus for decisions to forgo life-sustaining treatment does not assume
caring on the part of the surrogate but seems rather designed to guard
against chicanery."[14]

Problems with the Standard View

In the Prologue, alternative models of the ethics consultation process
were judged purely by pragmatic criteria: Which provides the most
fruitful conceptualization of the process, yielding the most insightful
questions? Views regarding the proper role of families in decision
making on behalf of incompetent persons, however, need to be
judged against a number of criteria. A theory such as the standard
view relies upon a mixture of factual and moral claims. It says some-

thing about the nature of families and the variety of family relationships: what families are commonly like, what claims they make, to what aberrations they are prone. It then takes this factual context and, identifying certain factors as ethically relevant, draws moral conclusions. This mixture of fact and value is evident in the fundamental assertion made by the standard view: Because of how they work, families legitimately claim a right to make decisions about the medical treatment of their incompetent members.

This kind of a mixed view requires examination on several levels: Does its description of families ring true? Does the average family function as the theory presumes, and does the aberrant family differ in the ways the theory predicts? Are the normative (ethical and legal) claims of the view coherent, understandable, and applicable? Do they yield acceptable results as applied to those cases frequently encountered? Is the logical connection between the factual claims and the ethical conclusions sound? Such an evaluation requires us to ask, in short: Does the standard view *describe* families accurately, and does it yield appropriate *prescriptions* for their participation in these decisions?

The standard view falls short on many of these evaluative criteria. I shall focus on only three of its shortcomings:

1. The way in which the standard view treats family conflict of interest
2. The standard view's beliefs about why families have a legitimate claim to make medical decisions
3. The actual moral claims made by families who wish their voices heard on these matters

Familial Conflict of Interest in the Standard View

As has been made clear, there is a strong tendency, in applying the standard view, to concentrate upon the prospect of family conflict of interest. Specifically, the standard view seems to foster a pervasive fear that families may choose that treatment that best serves their own interests, rather than those of their incompetent family member.

Family members themselves (a class that, one way or the other, includes most of us!) might reasonably take umbrage at such allegations—as a matter for repeated emphasis, theoretical elaboration, and routine practical suspicion, rather than as an occasionally well-grounded concern. What, after all, is the concrete reality behind this abstract discussion? A mother and father discussing proposed surgery for a handicapped child; a daughter struggling with the proposal that her demented mother be moved from her apartment to a skilled nursing facility; Mr. C, with growing fears regarding his own health at his advanced years, searching for a way to care for his psychotic son now and in years to come.

I have no doubt that in some such situations families take the easy way out for themselves, at the expense of the well-being of the patient; I have been involved in some such consultations. How often do they occur? I am aware of no studies addressing this question. But in my experience—very biased, to be sure, given the way in which I become involved in consultation—they are very rare, far too uncommon to deserve the attention the problem of family conflict of interest has received.

Why, then, does the standard view emphasize this problem as more suited to a television movie-of-the-week story conference than to a bioethics conference? First, because we can easily misidentify those cases in which there is a *confusion* of interests with those in which there exists a genuine *conflict*. Exciting clinical ethical cases usually possess an element of conflict between some health care providers and patients or their surrogates. Doctors, nurses, social workers—all consider themselves reasonable people and wonder why families resist their reasonable proposals. The only interest these health care workers have in their patients, they believe, is medical well-being. It is a small step from that to the presumption that other interests must be operating upon families who have reached different conclusions.

Often embroiled in such disputes through the consultation process, I have frequently shared a doctor's frustration in trying to "get through" to a family that is being "difficult." Yet before accusing families of being in a conflict of interest that should disqualify their participation, we should be convinced that the families agree that the doctor's recommendation is in the patient's best interest but resist it because it is contradictory to their own. I usually see different scenes: families that simply don't believe the doctor's diagnosis or prognosis or otherwise mistrust the doctor's competence, families that believe there are further choices that have not been presented to them, families that have been intellectually and emotionally burned out by being assaulted with unfamiliar terms and horrible options, and, yes, families that understand that for them the choice presented as medically clear-cut will mean further months or years of turmoil. Rarely is only one of these conditions present. Rarely can an outsider confidently claim that one specific circumstance was of decisive importance in generating the disagreement between family and hospital staff. As long as our notion of "family conflict of interest" remains fuzzy, however, it is almost always possible for the health care provider to claim its presence and, using the standard view, seek to disenfranchise an obstinate family.

Familial Conflict of Interest: Definitions and Double Binds

This leads us to a second, more fundamental problem. The standard view requires us to recognize when families are in conflict of interest and react appropriately. But do we even understand what this concept *means*? Karl Popper has argued that scientific proposals are more frequently meaningless because they explain too much, rather than too little.[15] For a theory to be meaningful it must be, in his words, falsifiable: We must be able to describe those experiments that would prove that the theory is mistaken, and if the theory will yield to no counterexamples, it must be dismissed as vacuous. The points made here suggest that this is true of the standard view as well.

At the heart of the standard view, and its understanding of family conflict of interest, lurks a series of catch-22s. Families gain the right to decide about medical treatment because of their closeness; families lose the right to decide because of a conflict of interest for that same reason, because the very definition of a close family is one in which whatever happens to each happens to all.

That is the foundational double bind; from it, many different ramifications are possible. For example: Families in general have a right to make these decisions because of their deep emotional investment in the patient, but *this* family should be forbidden to decide because their decisions are based upon emotion rather than reason. On the other hand, *that* family has no right to decide because they have failed to display the ordinary emotional attachments a family should exhibit. Then, of course, there is that *other* family: They are attached, but they are only acting out of guilt.

These bizarre, unanswerable charges of conflict and disqualification are not only made by outsiders. One scenario I have witnessed repeatedly involves conflict between an elderly patient's daughter and son. The daughter, who lives nearby and has been her parent's primary caregiver for the past several years of deterioration, wishes the health care team to preserve her parent's dignity by palliating symptoms and stopping progressively futile aggressive treatments. The son, who lives far away and has been an infrequent visitor, arrives at the sickbed, is shocked at his parent's condition, and immediately demands that "everything possible" be done. The son declares that his sister is asking for treatment to be withheld because she is worn out caring for the parent; the daughter counterclaims that the son's unreasonable posture is caused by his feelings of guilt that he has failed so badly at caring for his parent.

Within the law itself we can see the same damned-if-you-do, damned-if-you-don't approach. The case of *In re* Spring (see endnote 10), noted earlier, stands as authority for the proposition that a family's involvement in a treatment decision can be disqualified because its financial responsibility for the patient's care might lead family members to refuse treatment.[16] And yet, three years later, a Florida District Court of Appeals was faced with the question of whether the father of an adult, intellectually disabled woman has the authority to grant consent to treatment if he has not been legally appointed as guardian to the patient. The court decided in the affirmative; the father has that authority because he owes a continuing legal responsibility to financially support an adult incompetent child.[17]

The Family as a Decision-Making Unit: Hardwig's Alternative Approach

What has gone so wrong? The standard view has misconstrued ordinary, reasonable family relationships in a fundamental way, applying to them a model of conflict of interest drawn from (and better applied to) matters like business law. Any genuine family lives by creating an intricate web of interrelations between its members; the better the family, the more inextricably are its members bound. To look at normal family interactions and decisions and to see in them conflicts of interest is the sort of reaction a Martian would have—the same Martian who sees someone watching a television soap opera and accuses that person of eavesdropping.

The recognition that the standard view radically misunderstands family interactions is the central insight underlying a growing, alternative view of the family role in treatment decisions for incompetent patients. Taking off from the absurdity that the fact of family interest in the decision is treated by this view as a *disqualification,* John Hardwig has argued precisely the opposite proposition: He favors decision making by families despite the fact that these decisions will regularly be opposed to the best interests of patients—indeed, because of that very fact, and whether or not the patient acknowledges the weightiness of these contrary interests, as shown in these excerpts:

> To what extent can the patient's family legitimately be asked or required to sacrifice their interests so that the patient can have the treatment he or she wants? . . . Indeed, in many cases family members have a greater interest than the patient in which treatment option is exercised. In such cases, the interests of family members ought to *override* those of the patient. . . . I would argue that we must build our theory of medical ethics on the presumption of equality: the interests of patients and family members are morally to be weighed equally; medical and nonmedical interests of the same magnitude deserve equal consideration in making treatment decisions. Like any other moral presumption, this one can, perhaps, be defeated in some cases. But the burden of proof will always be on those who would advocate special consideration for any family member's interests, including those of the ill. . . . Some patients, motivated by a deep and abiding con-

cern for the well-being of their families, will undoubtedly consider the interests of other family members. For these patients, the interests of their family are *part* of their interests. But not all patients will feel this way. And the interests of family members are not relevant *if* and *because* the patient wants to consider them; they are not relevant because they are part of the patient's interests. They are relevant *whether or not* the patient is inclined to consider them.[18]

Between Realism and Cynicism: Roles Families Really Play

For some, this idea, grounded in a rejection of the standard view's unreal understanding of family conflict, has a more positive point to make: a vision of the family as an interdependent, organic unit, in which decisions about a patient's care are really decisions about the family. That concept, with some affinity to the philosophy of practice held by some family doctors,[19] is itself deeply flawed; for surely we can intelligibly argue, in particular circumstances, about whether or not a family decision does reflect a conflict of interest. For others, like Hardwig himself, the view to the contrary insists upon the reality of conflict of interest and an egalitarian perspective that the interests of nonpatients (family members) must count as equal to those of patients themselves. But this kind of universal concern is found in no other social transaction or institution (save, perhaps, certain views of social work). While the interests of my family are deeply affected when I decide to buy a house or take a vacation, this is of no concern to my real estate or travel agent. While it may represent an alternative social arrangement for health care, Hardwig's view implies the destruction, rather than reconstruction, of the ethics of medical practice: "If we retain the traditional ethic of fidelity to the interests of the patient, the physician should excuse herself from making treatment decisions that will affect the lives of the family on grounds of a moral conflict of interest, for she is a one-sided advocate."[20]

But finally, and paradoxically (for a view that began with a critique of how the standard view ignores or mistreats the interests of families), Hardwig's view misrepresents the way in which family interests are generally constructed and intertwined. Consider in this regard the paradoxes associated with the following excerpt from a case consultation.

ETHICS CONSULTATION:
PROLONGING TREATMENT AND LITIGATION

Mrs. W, a woman in her late twenties (and the mother of small children), was the victim of an anesthetic accident while undergoing a routine elective operation. She was deprived of oxygen for more than six minutes. She is now presumed to be in a persistent vegetative state, with massive-to-total destruction of her cerebral cortex caused by anoxia. Her family insists upon Mrs. W's receiving all life-prolonging measures, including cardiopulmonary resuscitation and artificial ventilation, as and when they might be needed.

The family has begun a multimillion-dollar malpractice lawsuit. Canadian courts usually provide much higher awards to living victims of malpractice than to the families of dead victims who lodge suits of wrongful death. Some staff have raised the possibility that the family's insistence upon Mrs. W's receiving any and all possible life-prolonging treatments is grounded in their interest in maximizing the monetary damages they may be awarded.

I spent a great deal of time thinking about this case.[21] Discussing it with an erstwhile colleague with a legal background, her reaction was that the family is in a clear conflict of interest, and the hospital should therefore seek to have decision-making power taken from the family and vested in a court representative.

That is an intelligible claim, and I could imagine circumstances in which it would be true. If, for example, the treatment the family wanted Mrs. W to undergo would cause her pain or discomfort, or if Mrs. W had left instructions in a living will asking that she not be treated under these circumstances, my colleague would have been right.

In this instance, however, I felt certain this colleague was wrong, for reasons that bring us to the second fundamental challenge to the standard view of the role of families. Let us assume for the sake of argument that my colleague was right and that the family's treatment demands were based upon their financial hopes from this litigation. My legal colleague was nonetheless wrong because the treatment the family demanded, invasive as it may be, could not cause Mrs. W pain or in any other objective way be contrary to her best interests. With the profound neurological damage she had suffered, Mrs. W was beyond feeling hurt or helped. And my colleague was wrong because, in the absence of a medical directive or living will to the contrary, the family was justified in assuming that their instructions are precisely what Mrs. W would herself have demanded had she been competent to answer the question. As the mother of a bereft husband and minor children in need of attention and care, it is reasonable to assume that Mrs. W would have agreed to being subjected to life-prolonging measures simply to make the lives of her family better.

This reinforces my claim that a family decision made in a confusion of interest does not constitute a conflict of interest. In good families, the interest of each is connected with the interest of all, as this mother's best interest might have required that her family's needs be securely satisfied. At the same time, this raises the question of whether families are generally good and reliable judges of what their (now-incompetent) family members would have wanted; this is the second crucial, but questionable, claim made by the standard view.

Families as Proxies in the Standard View

As discussed earlier, the standard view nominates families as decision makers for incompetent members because families are presumed to know, to care about, and to appropriately serve the best interests and preferences (present, previous, or imputed) of the patient in question. These abilities qualify families to serve as proxies whether the goal in reaching decisions for incompetent persons is to serve their best interests or to act as they would have directed had they been capable of considering and expressing a choice. Are these presumptions warranted?

Best Interests and Substituted Judgment:
Are Families Skillful Decision Makers?

In the absence of any evidence that family members consistently disregard the patient's own interest in favor of seeking their own, conflicting good, I see no reason to doubt that family members are good "best-interests" proxies. But this basis for family authority is nonetheless weak, for the family is certainly not the *only* group that can serve this role, nor are they necessarily the *best-equipped* for it. At least for strictly medical decisions, the doctors, nurses, and other health care providers caring for the patient have equally good or better claims of being able to judge the course of treatment that will best serve the patient. (Social workers will often make the same claim regarding broader, more custodial decisions.) The experience of others may confirm my own that, over time, given sufficient education about the implications of the choice and opportunity to discuss it, most families come to agree with well-considered medical recommendations. That shows that families are not *disqualified* under a best-interests criterion, however, not that the criterion requires that we choose families to play the role of proxy decision maker.

As providers of "substituted judgment"—the decision the patient would have given had he or she been competent—families are in an even weaker position. The family, in playing this role, should be bringing to bear the best evidence possible: the patient's solemn, written statement of preferences (living will) if available; failing in that, the patient's previously expressed, coherent, and relevant statement of preferences ("If I should ever become depressed, I would not want to languish for months waiting for drugs to start working; I would want you to start electroconvulsive therapy right away"). If that too is absent, the family should be extrapolating from the patient's previous lifestyle and values. In each case, the family should be judging as the patient would have judged and should avoid intruding their own values and preferences.

Informally, we have long been aware that families often resist or evade this act of imagination. Time and again, when a doctor or ethics consultant asks a wife acting as a proxy whether this is what her husband would have wanted, she responds, "Of course he would! It's the only reasonable thing to do! He would have to be crazy not to!" This confident claim arises as often in very difficult borderline situations of medical choice as it does in those that are indeed clear-cut. I have been much more impressed with the family's ability to provide a substituted judgment in the rare cases when they propose a decision that they themselves emphasize they dislike ("But it's what she would have wanted") than in the very common cases in which there is an eerie coincidence between what the family has decided it wants and what they claim the patient would have wanted. (Commonly, the family changes its mind with the passage of time, without disturbing the prearranged harmony between what they choose and what they feel the patient would have chosen.)

The Lessons of Research: Families as Proxy Decision Makers

This informal sense has been confirmed recently with the creation of a booming cottage industry investigating family ability to serve this role. Linda and Ezekiel Emanuel, two of the most assiduous investigators of this phenomenon, sum up the findings:

> For a proxy to carry out the patient's wishes, several things must happen. First, patients must designate a proxy. Then they must discuss their treatment preferences with the proxy. Next, the proxy must understand the patient's preferences, and finally, the proxy must make the same choices as the patient would have. The existing research suggests that these events are not taking place very well. . . . [M]any studies have indicated that concordance between patient and proxy is far from perfect.[22]

Much of this literature shares a basic structure. One population of subjects is chosen to act as "the patient" and is presented with a variety of choices associated with scenarios set out by the investigators. (For example: If you were ill with advanced cancer, and no longer capable of speaking for yourself, and had failed to respond to chemotherapy the last time it was tried, would you want it tried again anyway? If your heart stopped beating under those circumstances, would you want it restarted? etc.) Family members of the group acting as "the patient" are presented with the same scenarios but are cautioned to decide as "the patient" would have decided.

Despite this common structure, the details differ between studies. Some investigators might choose as "patients" a group with diverse demographic characteristics, while others will choose a group of elderly persons more likely to face the posited scenarios soon; yet others have studied persons who are actually hospitalized at the time of the study, whether or not actually facing the posited scenarios. Some have studied in detail a very small number of "patients"; others, via questionnaire, a much larger group. Some have tried to ascertain whether subjects actually comprehended the choices presented; others have not. Ancillary questions were studied by some, but not all, of these studies. For example: Has there been previous discussion between family members over such matters? Do you think the family proxy will "get it right" and so instruct the doctors? The diversity of these studies is useful because there is no obvious "right way" to study this question.

Overall, as Linda and Ezekiel Emanuel note, the results are not reassuring. The conclusion of one of the better studies is quite representative: "Our results suggest that the recommended approach to medical decisions in patients of diminished capacity—surrogates using substituted judgment—may be seriously flawed."[23] In that study of seventy chronically ill (but not demented) geriatric patients, the scenarios asked whether cardiopulmonary resuscitation should be attempted if needed under the subject's current state of health, as well as under a state in which the patient had grown demented to the point of no longer recognizing family and friends. The responses of these subjects were compared to what the subjects' family proxy (the family member chosen by the subject as the preferred decision maker) and primary care physicians thought the subjects wanted or would want. Despite the fact that most "patients" had not discussed these matters previously with their family members (84%) or doctors (93%), most were confident these proxies could accurately predict their wishes (doctor: 90%; family member: 87%). The confidence was misplaced: Doctors' predictions are described as being no better than chance, and even the proportion of agreement between family members and patients was not high enough to surpass the usual measure (kappa > 0.40) applied to statistically ensure greater-than-chance agreement.

The Standard View and Family Roles: A Case Study

Given this evidence, the discrediting of the standard view is as a theoretical matter complete. Before departing from it, however, there is one last—and perhaps most crucial—test to perform: the effect that the standard view may have upon a clinical ethical issue. The following excerpt describes a case that I found almost uniquely repugnant, although—because!—its result was satisfactory to adherents of the standard view. A proper consideration of this case may both suggest what is fundamentally wrong with that view, and what should replace it.

ETHICS CONSULTATION:
OLD FAMILY SECRET—A MODERN GOTHIC STORY

Mrs. A, a woman in her eighties, has been a resident of a psychiatric hospital in _____ since the early 1940s. Following an initial diagnosis of postpartum depression, she has been variously described as suffering from schizophrenia, schizo-affective disorder, and other similar disorders, all with "schizo" in them. She has been on antipsychotic medications for many years, practically since their introduction into clinical use. She recently had an episode of chest pain that was probably an ischemic event, and her health is worsening. She seems unlikely to live for very long.

Proxy consent (and refusal) has been provided on her behalf by her niece, who is now refusing aggressive measures (which were said in her chart to be contraindicated "because of her underlying condition," by which is presumably meant psychiatric condition—a statement that may be invidiously discriminatory or may simply represent an egregious misstatement of a medical conclusion reasonable on other, unstated grounds). It doesn't appear this niece has seen her aunt more than, at most, very occasionally. Throughout this critical episode the record indicates that she has spoken with staff but not necessarily met with and spoken with Mrs. A herself.

Mrs. A has a daughter in her fifties living in a nearby city. She wants to see her daughter. Also, a treating psychiatrist, who disagrees with the niece's decision to withhold treatment from Mrs. A, thinks the daughter should be contacted to serve as Mrs. A's proxy decision maker. The problem is that the daughter does not know where her mother is, nor indeed that she is alive. Two different stories have surfaced, and it was not clear to my informant which is correct. In one version, the mother was admitted to the psychiatric hospital when her daughter was three years old, in the other, when she was eleven; in one version, the daughter was told her mother had abandoned the family; in the other, that her mother had died.

Mrs. A's husband had concealed the truth from his daughter for many years. When he died, in 1977, he left instructions that the secret be kept from his daughter in perpetuity. He vested decision making over Mrs. A's purse and person in his sister; in the event of his sister's death, which subsequently transpired, in his sister's daughter, i.e., the niece. The niece is adamant that the daughter not be notified of her mother's situation and has stated that this information would devastate her and probably cause her to be institutionalized as well.

The presenting questions concerned the choice of a proxy decision maker and the underlying ethics of revelation or continued concealment in this situation. The issue is seen by the hospital in which Mrs. A is confined as a deep and difficult ethical dilemma. A meeting of that hospital's ethics committee is to be held on Monday, which my informant will be attending.

I could be of little assistance in helping explain how this case is a dilemma rather than an ethical outrage: I found the story deeply, almost uniquely, revolting.

I can see no moral basis for respecting Mr. A's wish to keep the secret and to vest authority over his wife in a sister or niece. I do not believe such an instruction can have legal force either, and if I am right in that belief, the attorney involved in drafting these instructions should have his conduct reviewed by the bar for possibly violating professional legal ethics. Mrs. A was not chattel, bric-à-brac, to be disposed of by her husband.

The issue of choice of medical treatment I thought was likely to prove to be a red herring. From the description provided of Mrs. A's medical condition, brief as it was, it seemed probable that aggressive treatment would be futile, in the sense that when Mrs. A becomes dependent upon intensive care she would be so deteriorated as to not survive to discharge from the ICU. This case has not, however, been reviewed up to this point by anyone with the appropriate medical expertise. I suggested that the chart should be reviewed by an intensive care specialist, who should attend the ethics committee meeting or at least provide input regarding whether there is a genuine possibility of successful treatment.

The real question concerns notification of the daughter. I consider this question to be of great importance, going beyond the instrumental value associated with this notification. Telling, and knowing, the truth in this case is a privilege, and perhaps a duty. Mrs. A is (prima facie) entitled to see her daughter and to say goodbye; she may be duty-bound to do that as well, and her desire to fulfill this duty should not be frustrated. The daughter is entitled, and perhaps duty-bound, to know the truth as well. Even our anomic, secular society recognizes duties back and forth between mothers and children.

The information will probably be difficult to deal with, as insight in life is often difficult. (It might, on the other hand, in fact be a relief, if the daughter finds out that she was not rejected or abandoned by her mother.) Even granted difficulty, that should not in itself be a decisive consideration. The niece should, however, be questioned regarding the basis of her belief that the daughter would react to this news by having a psychotic breakdown. (It is barely possible that this belief is well-grounded.) In addition, perhaps the daughter's personal physician could be contacted confidentially and asked his/her view of her probable reaction. I am not sure what could be learned from the niece or physician that would justify withholding this information, but I would not rule out the possibility a priori. Certainly, there is a heavy burden of proof against the view that the secret should still be kept. My informant also pointed out that in the end the secret must come out. Another person now aware of the issue is a government official who deals with trusts and inheritance. He confirmed that Mrs. A has an estate. He finds the case ethically troubling, but feels he has no options. After Mrs. A's death, when her estate devolves to her daughter, the daughter must discover both the truth and the fact that she had been kept in the dark these many years. Given that fact, it seems to me virtually certain that, however difficult it will be for the daughter to deal with the truth about her mother, her chances of dealing with this successfully will be enhanced by learning of her mother while there is still a chance to see and speak with her, and to come to terms with the burden of lies and secrecy laid down by the years.

The possibility of adverse concealment should be recognized. The hospital may see this as a difficult ethical dilemma because they want to continue the concealment so the daughter does not sue them for keeping from her the truth—as she may be right to do. The niece may wish to keep the secret because she has designs upon Mrs. A's estate. Stranger, and more vicious, motives have been known to operate. The entire story has an abhorrent, Faulknerian miasma about it. At the time of the story's beginning, it was not unknown for husbands to seek to have their difficult and disobedient wives undergo coercive and excessive psychiatric treatment, culminating in the wives' psychic collapse. But we do not need recourse to these hypotheses to conclude that there is almost certainly a duty to break the chain of silence and deceit so that a family might be reunited in the face of pending separation by death.

The following week, the hospital's ethics committee met. They were joined by a consultant in clinical ethics, whose services were engaged ad hoc for the purpose of attending this meeting and assisting the hospital with this problem. With the concurrence of this consultant, the committee decided that the niece is the appropriate decision maker. In principle, they said, ethically, proxy choice is vested in a relative because of one or both of two factors: A near relative is likely to be bound by affection and thus can be trusted to act in the patient's best interests, or the relative is likely to be apprised of the patient's values or wishes regarding treatment. While the niece was far from perfect from these points of view, she nonetheless was held by them to be a more satisfactory proxy than the daughter.

My informant, fortified with our discussion, argued to the contrary and lost; this person's role was too peripheral and his credibility too low to sway the committee. I expressed my own desire to pursue this further. The result was so repugnant, and the role played by the consultant who had been hired so damaging to my profession, that I thought it worthwhile to assume the risk of the lawsuit that might ensue over my disclosure of the confidential information I had received. My informant, however, refused me permission to do this, fearing the political consequences to his own position.[24]

A Family Duty

The standard view, despite its widespread appeal and initial plausibility, is simply unacceptable. It was based upon elements that we have examined and found wanting: Families, (1) purged of conflict of interest, (2) claim the right to render decisions about the medical care of their incompetent members, based upon their acquaintance with (3) the best interest of the patient and (4) the patient's preferences. With the problems noted with Hardwig's alternative view, however, how should we understand and reconstruct the role of the family?

Family Decision Making: Right or Duty?

I believe the key lies in examining the standard view's second premise, hitherto unquestioned: Families *claim the right* to make these decisions. Within our legal system, of course, a claimant seeking the court's attention must come armed with a right. In our courts, families must speak the language of rights. But in considering the role, and claim, of families to decide, we should not allow the moral point of view to be co-opted by legal considerations. Very few of these cases will end up in court; even serious conflicts will usually be resolved within the clinical setting, and it is that setting that must remain our chief concern. "Families claim the right": Is that an accurate understanding of the role that families claim, or is it rather a clumsy, legalistic misconstrual of the moral basis of the claim of families to decide about the care of their incompetent members?

The best and most natural way of describing the claim of families speaks instead the language of duty: Families understand that it is their obligation to see to, and decide about, this patient's medical care, as it is their obligation to feed, and clothe, and comfort, and succor. This duty of medical decision making is continuous with all the other obligations owed to a family member who is unable to care for herself.

The studies that described how poorly families perform when trying to predict the medical preferences of incompetent persons are disturbing for a number of reasons. However, if family involvement in decision making is understood as a claim of duty rather than a right, although this lack of communication may represent a failing in families, it in no way undercuts the normative basis for their involvement in these decisions. As Joanne Lynn noted,

> I, and surely some other patients, prefer family choice over the opportunity to make our own choices in advance. The patient himself or herself may well judge the family's efforts less harshly than he or she would judge his or her own decisions made in advance or by the professional caregivers. I have had a number of seriously ill patients say that their next of kin will attend to some choice if it comes up. When challenged with the possibility that the next of kin might decide in a way that was not what the patient would have chosen, the patient would kindly calm my concern with the observation that such an error would not be very important.[25]

The Patient's View of the Role of the Family
in Medical Decision Making

Dallas High has carefully listened to and written about the reasons why elderly persons in his region (the southern United States) so commonly state their preference for a family decision maker in the event that they should become incompetent to decide on their own behalf. His informants provide a variety of reasons for this, despite suggestions that a non–family member would do better:

> A 70-yr-old woman: "I think it should be my husband and two children. And, of course, if he's not living then the two children, because they are the ones who would have to see after me."
>
> A 77-yr-old widow, asked whether friends or a doctor or lawyer would qualify as surrogates: "No one else. Don't need them. Just use my girls. What did I raise them for?"
>
> A 71-yr-old divorcee, defying geography, insists that her children should make these decisions in spite of the fact that none lives within 400 miles of her: "They don't live here, but they would get together and decide; I am sure."
>
> Acknowledging the possibility of conflict among the children, one other informant says: "But I feel that they're as capable of, let's say, fighting it out between 'em, and working it out, as I am now of saying who should do what."[26]

Think of the adult children of a father with advancing dementia: They seek out an appropriate facility for him to live in, asking questions, raising issues, investigating responses and alternatives, and raising a ruckus when needed. When a doctor comes along with a new proposal for treatment, should they do any less?

In speaking with them about their own moral understanding, without exception, every adult child caring for an elderly, frail parent has described this to me as a duty. The language of obligations is, in that setting, intuitively right. The same would apply, I believe, in other instances of caring for incompetent adults: a husband describing the basis of his claim to decide treatment for his wife, muted by stroke; a sibling caring for a brother with advanced Huntington's disease.

To some, this language of duty does not capture well the claim of a parent vis-à-vis a minor child; to them, it is more natural to describe this as the right to care for the child. I believe this is the result of a confusion. We tend to equate caring for adults with duty in part because of its onerous nature, and we resist it with respect to children because of the joy associated with fulfilling that duty. But it is a mistake to confuse these in this way; a person may be unhappy at the freedom of choice implied by a right. And one whose life is lived for duty finds his or her happiness in its fulfillment: The Psalmist writes, "I rejoice in Your words as one who has found great treasure."[27] This theme, naturally enough, permeates Jewish literature. One illustrative story: At the time of the Roman persecutions, the teaching of the Law was punishable by death. The Talmud records a debate among the rabbis over how to react to the decree: one side argued that for the present, it would be prudent to disobey the decree in secret, if at all. The leader of the other side was Rabbi Akiva, whose argument was suggested to him by his wife, Rachel: "Go and tell the rabbis," she said, "that even more than the calf wishes to suck does the cow need to suckle."

Once the question of who will speak for the voiceless reaches a North American court, the claim must be reformulated as a right rather than a duty. This is easily done. A principle of moral logic has it that "ought implies can": A person could not be duty-bound to perform some action unless that person is capable of its performance; this capability entails legal, as well as physical, ability. By this logic, the reason for the court to grant a right (a legal power) is so that a duty may be satisfied. But even if it ultimately results in the recognition of a right to decide, it remains important to realize that the primordial basis of the family's claim to a role—their own understanding of why they seek involvement—is duty. This comes out clearly in George Fletcher's discussion of one celebrated custody case, in which Mary Beth Whitehead, who had borne a child for another couple (pursuant to a so-called surrogate-mother contract), attempted to retain legal custody of Baby M:

The New Jersey Supreme Court adopted a peculiar way of talking about a mother's claim to care for her own child. The question was supposedly one of the mother's "right to the companionship of her child" [footnote omitted]. American lawyers and judges commonly phrase every issue as an expression of individual rights, but I take it that the dominant thought motivating mothers like Mary Beth Whitehead is not the notion of right but of duty. The mother of Baby M felt compelled to care for her offspring.[28]

Judaism on Duties of Children to Parents: Respectful Service and Reverent Obedience

I wish to turn now to a Jewish perspective, a tradition that allows us to consider duties directly and unashamedly, without such clumsy expediencies as a translation to "rights" language. Compare the passage by Fletcher with the following discussion of custody law by the Israeli rabbinate:

> Problems concerning the contact between the child and his parents are questions of the child's rights and his good, but not of the rights of the father or the rights of the mother. Rights such as these [latter] do not exist at all. . . . The Jewish laws [halakhot] regarding the custody of children are not laws involving the parents' good, but rather laws involving the good of children; the son or daughter is not a material object over which parents may claim rights. *No parental rights are here present, but only duties incumbent upon them, that render them duty-bound to raise and educate their children.*[29]

The contrast between the Jewish legal view, centered on duty, and that with which we are familiar, centered upon rights, is pervasive. Within our legal system, to possess a legal personality is to be a rights-possessor. Therefore, the milestones whereby a child reaches the age of maturity and joins the legal community are marked with the acquisition of rights: to drive, to drink, to leave home, to get married, to vote, and so forth. Within the Jewish legal system, to be a legal person is to be a duty-possessor. The child entering the community is called a *bar-mitzva* or *bat-mitzva*, literally, "a son or daughter of commandments," one who is now the object of legal obligations.[30]

The Biblical Basis for a Family Role

What specific duty is asserted by the family, and how do its claims differ from (or influence the construal of resulting) claims of right? As was suggested in the earlier case of placement for a demented parent, the duty of rendering medical decisions is continuous with, or an extension of, a general duty upon the family to care for its members who cannot care for themselves. I will for the remainder of this chapter, however, concentrate on the specific issue of adult children claiming a role in medical decision making regarding their incompetent parent.

Within a Jewish understanding, of course, that issue involves several specific biblical injunctions, each with its own nuance of concern, including:

> Each of you shall fear his mother and father, and guard my Sabbaths; I am G-d.[31]

> One who strikes his father and mother shall surely die. One who curses his father and mother shall surely die.[32]

Above all looms the Fifth Commandment:

> Honor your father and your mother; so that your days may be lengthened upon the land that G-d your L-rd gives to you.[33]

Rabbinic Interpretation: Duty in Concrete Understanding

The Jewish (and, especially, talmudic) manner of describing and prescribing duty most typically involves the furnishing of specific, concrete instantiations of the duties in question. These paradigm cases are then further analyzed by examining their distinctive normative characteristics. The talmudic definition of the Fifth Commandment is exemplary in this regard:

> What is "honoring"? Causes to eat and to drink, clothes and covers, brings in and brings out [ma'akhil umashke, malbish um'khase, makhnis umotzi].[34]

This particular concretization of the obligation subsumes the following points:

- The duty must be manifest through behavior, and not— or not only—through attitude or emotional attachment.
- The child is commanded, *inter alia,* to personally serve the parent, to provide the parent's basic physical needs: food, water, clothing, transportation. In this way, everyday filial interaction is invested with dutiful solemnity (and so, in Judaism's religious worldview, is sanctified).
- These instantiations share a characteristic form of talmudic ambiguity. How, precisely, does one cause a parent to eat? The answer will depend upon the condition and need of the parent and will vary as the parent's circumstances of life change; yet, while the expression of the duty will vary, its essential content will remain unchanged.

Think of a child and parent through the years. The young son accompanies his mother shopping, and "helps": He has caused her to eat. In early adulthood, flush with his first paycheck, he takes her out for a restaurant meal. The years pass, she is widowed and grows frail: He arranges for a homemaker to visit. She suffers a stroke and needs to be fed carefully by hand. Finally, she loses the ability to swallow, and he is faced with a decision to have her fed by tube. "Causes to eat": The duty to honor parents is the red thread running through, and binding together, these events and circumstances; it is that which explains the role the son seeks to fulfill in medical decision making concerning his incompetent parent.

Positive Claims in a Regime of Duty

I had earlier discussed some differences between an ethics consultation grounded in a model of duty and one based upon rights: the differences in the approach of those models to conflict, to the nature of an acceptable resolution, to the question of who participates in a discussion and in what way. All these differences hold true when considering whether the basis of family participation in decision making for incompetent members is grounded in their right or in their duty. In discussing the Jewish understanding of what it means to "honor" a parent, however, another facet of the difference between these regimes is revealed. The regime of rights, predicated upon the autonomy of individuals, is comfortable handling its members' negative claims, claims to be let alone, but has trouble accommodating positive claims, to assistance and succor. The regime of duties is not limited in that way; as Robert Cover puts it,

> The jurisprudence of rights has proved singularly weak in providing for the material guarantees of life and dignity flowing from the community to the individual. While we may talk of the right to medical care, the right to subsistence, the right to an education, we are constantly met by the realization that such rhetorical tropes are empty in a way that the right to freedom of expression or the right to due process are not. When the issue is restraint upon power it is intelligible to simply state the principle of restraint. . . . However, the "right to an education" is not even an intelligible principle unless we know to whom it is addressed. Taken alone it only speaks to a need. A distributional premise is missing which can only be supplied through a principle of "obligation.". . . [Yet in Judaism, which has had unparalleled access to education,] it is striking that the Jewish legal materials never speak of the right or entitlement of the child to an education. Rather, they speak of the obligation incumbent upon various providers to make the education available. It is a *mitzvah* for a father to educate his son, or grandson. It is a *mitzvah* for a teacher under certain circumstances to teach even without remuneration.[35]

Four Expressions of Filial Obligation

Jewish law recognizes a general category of "honoring" parents, *kibud av v'em,* and within that category distinguishes diverse forms of obligation. Traditionally, the prohibition against harming a parent is treated separately from the positive obligations, *kibud* and *morah.* Because of the central significance of issues arising from the obligation not to harm a parent, however, I am including that in the discussion. For our purposes, we can distinguish four distinct filial obligations,[36] which are drawn from the verses presented earlier.[37]

1, 2. The prohibitions against striking (1) or denigrating (2) a parent, based upon the verses in Exodus, Chapter 21, extend beyond these narrow bounds. They also implicate obligations to prevent parents from experiencing pain (1) and indignity (2) respectively. These will be dealt with in the following section.

3. The obligation to "honor" *[kibud, l'khaved]* parents by providing for their physical needs is grounded in the Talmud's interpretation of the Fifth Commandment, cited earlier. (I will not here enter into the complicated question of when a child is required to undergo financial sacrifice on behalf of *kibud.*)

4. The obligation to "fear" (or stand in awe of; *morah*) the parent is expressed in the verse from Leviticus. The same talmudic passage cited earlier about "honor" defines "fear" in this way: "What constitutes 'fear'? He does not sit in his [parent's] place and does not speak in his stead and he does not contradict his statements." The Talmud connected these signs of formal respect and obedience to the injunction to "fear" of the parent, an expression that signifies subjugation of the will. The verse compelling this attitude toward parents, and that behavior which is appropriate to "fear," appears at the beginning of the "Chapter of Holiness," describing the solemn obligations imposed by a transcendent G-d. The term, its concept, and the context in which it appears all point in the same direction: the child's reverence of a parent as of a master, a ruler—and even, a Ruler[38]—and the behavior appropriate to that attitude, obedience.

First Category of Filial Obligation: The Claims of *Kibud*

A different relationship is invoked by "honor" itself, or rather *kibud,* a term that admits of no fully satisfactory English translation. *Kibud* in its origins relates to the Hebrew root *KBD,* meaning weighty, heavy, considerable. To provide *kibud* to parents therefore implies recognizing their importance, treating them as "weighty," avoiding behavior that takes them "lightly." At the same time, this form of "honor" is expressed by personal attention to the needs of the other; to grant *kibud* is in fact one Hebrew phrase for serving a meal to a guest. The single Hebrew concept of *kibud,* then, instantiates respectful and fitting service to the parent.

A language reflects a culture and its norms and crafts terms accordingly. It is no accident, then, that Hebrew offers these two words, *morah* and *kibud,* that each in their own way express dutiful attitudes and their corresponding behavior. The closest we might come to an English equivalent would be to call *kibud* "respectful service" and *morah* "reverent obedience." The stilted, artificial, awkward quality of these phrases is itself testimony to our culture's discomfort with them. Take, for example, *kibud,* as seen in the following case.

ETHICS CONSULTATION: MOTHER, DAUGHTER, CLSC

A ninety-two-year-old woman had been cared for at home by her daughter for the past eight years; the daughter is said to have made a deathbed promise to her father to tend to the woman. The patient was admitted with infection (probably pneumonia), which has now been cleared. She is ready for discharge, scheduled for tomorrow. However, she is not mobile and discharge evaluation has confirmed she is not "rehabilitable." In all respects, however, she has regained her "baseline of function," that is, the same level of ability she had prior to admission. Previously, her mobility was in any event restricted to the use of a walker in her apartment and its balcony.

Her daughter is described as "pathologically devoted." She has been by the mother's bedside day and night throughout this hospitalization, leaving only to nap for a few hours while some-one else stays with her. This daughter refuses to sign high-care nursing home long-term care papers for her mother; she wants to bring her back home. Dr. H agrees that with maximal com-munity and home care support this could be attempted safely. However, the CLSC (Centre Loisir et Santé Communitaire), the government agency that provides community and home nursing services, acting on the discharge evaluation of one of their social workers, refuses to provide this support. The agency has found that by their norms the mother is not functional enough to remain at home and insists that she must rather be placed in a skilled nursing facility. The patient herself is com-petent and wants to go home.

Under the circumstances, Dr. H feels that if this mother and daughter leave for home, they should first sign papers indi-cating discharge against medical advice. The staff have some concern that they may be liable in the event that the mother should leave and some misadventure befall her. I explained that they might instead want to be concerned about the liability they would incur on account of kidnapping or unlawfully confining this patient, insofar as that is what would be required to keep her in hospital or move her to a nursing facility against her competent directives. I further advised that in my judgment the government agency was acting in contradiction to its legislative and bureaucratic mandate by restricting the woman's options in this way (moreover, contrary to the discharging doctor's opin-ion). The law here guarantees a competent patient freedom of placement and freedom from attempts by the government or other parties to restrict, coerce, or circumvent that freedom.

This case is one among many raising issues about the discharge of frail elderly patients on which I have been consulted. I have spent a fair bit of time in those meetings talking about our local system for determining when people need institutional placement of one or an-other variety (foster home, skilled nursing facility, geriatric hospital, etc.). The assessment involves filling out a standard form in which numbers are assigned to various aspects of a person's condition: capacity to move around with or without assistance, ability to perform activities of daily living (such as toileting, bathing, care of fingernails and toenails), and so on. The numbers did not add up for this woman; on this scheme, she "belonged" in a nursing home.

Yet what we measure reflects social values and presuppositions as much as it does the condition of the patient. Obviously, there is much a daughter or son may provide at home that institutional care won't provide, but there are no boxes to tick off on the discharge form that reflect this fact. This is not because there is no way to quantify the more intangible benefits of being cared for at home by your child. One could, if one chose, quantify the estimated number of words spoken to a patient in the course of a day, or the amount of time it would take for the patient to adjust to her new surroundings. But our local system simply never bothered to include this information when constructing its rules about discharge planning.

Another factor the system fails to adequately consider is the nature of the daughter's involvement and claim. She is not claiming a "right," and there is no need to weigh her "rights" to be with her mother against her mother's "right" to safety. She wishes rather to fulfill a vow made at her father's deathbed; a duty, moreover, to which she is bound "by an oath made at Mount Sinai," in the rabbinic phrase: the duty of *kibud*, respectful service, to parents. Sometimes this duty is implicated directly, as in decisions about discharge of a parent. But it is equally implicated indirectly, when a son or daughter demands a role in determining the nature of care that a parent will receive in hospital, for the child may, as circumstances require, fulfill the duty to "cause to eat and cause to drink, take out and take in" directly or by proxy. By helping to ensure that an institution adequately attends to a parent's needs, the child's involvement in the care of a parent makes the institution act as the child's agent in fulfilling this duty. The daughter in this case has perhaps taken her obligation to saintly extremes, but certainly to describe her actions as "pathological devotion" says more about the speaker's values than about this daughter's.

Testing the Limits of *Kibud:*
Personal Service for a Demented Parent

There are many descriptions in the rabbinic literature of the nature and limits of what this *kibud* entails. We need to take care, in delineating the demands of duty, to distinguish that which is required from that which is ideal. This is not always easy, and this daughter's actions, exemplary as they may have been, for that very reason may not illuminate the demands of duty. It is not always possible for *kibud* to be expressed in the manner this daughter chose; it may not even always be wise. This is the question at the base of a dispute between the early medieval rabbis Rambam (Rabbi Moses ben Maimon, commonly known as Maimonides) and Ra'avad (Rabbi Avraham Ibn Da'ud). Rambam writes,

> One whose father or mother has become deranged *[nit'r'fa da'ato]* tries to behave with them according to their mental state until they should "receive mercy" [i.e., until they should either be healed or die]. But if it is impossible for him to bear this because of their excessive derangement, he should leave them and go his own way, and command others to treat them in that manner which is appropriate to them.[39]

Ra'avad protested: "This is an incorrect ruling; if he should leave them, to whom shall he command their care?" Most subsequent writers, however, accepted Rambam's view.[40] The question of whether and when a child's respectful service, *kibud,* may be rendered by arranging institutional placement for a demented parent is of course a common and excruciatingly difficult contemporary problem.

There are two ways of understanding Rambam's ruling, each of which suggests a different rationale for limiting the obligation of *kibud.* The first view is that Rambam's statement reflects the idea that *kibud* cannot be required at any and all costs to the child's welfare. Gerald Blidstein accordingly writes that it is clear that "the main consideration for Maimonides is the welfare of the son."[41]

According to this view, care of a demented parent comes to pose a conflict between the child's duty of respectful service and his own needs (or, if you like, his obligation to secure his own well-being). In this conflict, Rambam rules that the child's needs take priority. However, he is not absolved of his obligation to care for the parent: That obligation persists, but it is to be fulfilled indirectly, by placing the parent in the care of others.

By speaking of the child's own needs, of course, I do not mean the child's own mere preference or convenience. Rambam here may reflect a consistent view he had developed: that it is simply impossible for a sane person to dwell with one who has become deeply deranged. (I have seen no discussion of the source of this view, which may, however, have arisen from his experience as a physician.) We find this same view expressed in the context of the laws of divorce, which prevent a husband from divorcing a wife who has become mentally incompetent (see Section 3); Rambam writes,

> If she has become incompetent, he cannot expel her until she becomes healthy. . . . Therefore, he leaves her, and marries another, but he arranges for her food . . . for a sane person is incapable of living in a single house with those who are incompetent.[42]

A second approach was innovated by R Eli'ezer Waldenberg, in his response to a scholarly correspondent whose mother had apparently developed severe dementia with attendant agitation.[43] The doctors have instructed him to place his mother in restraints, and he asks R Waldenberg whether he is permitted to follow their orders. R Waldenberg, in reviewing the controversy following Rambam's ruling, emphasizes that both Ra'avad and those later authorities who criticized Rambam[44] had misquoted one crucial phrase of the ruling, namely, that the son commands others to treat his parents "in that manner which is appropriate to them." He understands the significance of this phrase as follows:

> When it is impossible for him [the son] to stay with them [the parents] because, due to their most extreme derangement, it is

necessary to deal with them in a forceful fashion, like tying them with ropes [i.e., restraining them] . . . : This, the son cannot do because of the Torah commandment incumbent upon him. It was of this that Maimonides wrote that "he should leave them, and command others to treat them as is appropriate for them"; which is to say, that others should treat them with the appropriate forceful measures that are made necessary by their insanity. . . . Therefore, in my view it is simple and obvious as a matter of law that the son is forbidden to tie up his mother to the chair on account of her insanity; but it is incumbent upon him to transfer her into the hands of others who will deal with her in this way if it is appropriate to her deranged condition, and necessary, in accordance with the relevant doctor's orders.[45]

In this second view, Rambam's ruling reflects not an exception to the child's duty of *kibud,* but rather the only means to fulfill it under these trying circumstances. The child is in that paradoxical situation wherein the "service" the parent requires is, from a certain viewpoint, inherently disrespectful.

There is, to be sure, room for controversy over whether restraints are overused in the impaired geriatric population and for ethical debate over what role they should play (if any),[46] as there is over such "forceful" measures as coerced psychiatric confinement and treatment. Unless one adopts the position that there are *never* circumstances that justify these interventions, however—something I am certainly not prepared to say—the adult child of a neurologically or psychiatrically impaired parent may at some point face this paradox.

Although I have posed this as a dispute between two understandings of Rambam, there is what may be a better reading. The views of Professor Blidstein and of R Waldenberg reflect the ambivalence and tension felt by adult children confronted with a medical recommendation for institutionalization or forced psychiatric treatment of an incompetent parent. Does one accede to this recommendation because, as R Waldenberg argues, that is what *kibud* calls for here, or does one agree because one has reached a personal breaking point and needs for the sake of one's own sanity to hand the problem of caring for a parent over to others?

Questions of placement of an impaired parent, and the care which that parent should receive, are true dilemmas of *kibud*. (And not only of parents; compare the earlier case of Ben.) As such, I do not find in Jewish sources a general and definitive resolution of these questions. Something will be lost no matter how the prdblem is resolved. What these sources do afford, however, is a framework of duty within which to consider these problems and a language we may use to discuss them.

Second Category of Filial Obligation: *Morah*

The second norm for honoring parents is *morah,* reverent obedience. It is this category that is invoked in cases associated with the fulfillment of any prior instructions on medical care an incompetent patient had provided, including so-called living wills. When such instructions are available, family members are generally relieved that the burden of decision making has been lifted from them: Their duty of *morah* is clear. But not all instructions are clear, nor do all family members see this in the same way.

ETHICS CONSULTATION: SOME PATIENTS ARE LOCKED IN; MAYBE SOME RELATIVES SHOULD BE LOCKED OUT

Mr. L is an Ashkenazic Jewish man, about eighty years old, with a variety of preexisting medical conditions. In January of this year, in Florida, he was treated for a stroke and released. Other indications are that he's had a series of mild strokes. Last month, he had another major stroke in northern New York State and came back to Montreal for treatment, begun at another hospital and transferred for mysterious reasons to our own.

The CT scan has confirmed a stroke in the brain stem that has conserved his ability to breathe. His current status is grim. On a couple of occasions he may have been volitionally moving his eyes or eyelids. He is now either permanently comatose or unconscious and in a locked-in state [i.e., totally paralyzed]. If he "improves" any further, it would be to a conscious locked-in state with an irreversible etiology. He has to date been treated quite aggressively. A tube has been left in for care of the airway. Dr. T had noted in the chart that he is henceforward to receive primarily palliative measures. He has no infection or other active condition at this time.

The discussion of his treatment was held with three sons (to be called here Shimon, Levi, and Yehuda) and one daughter (Dina); a second daughter is in Vancouver. The discussion was precipitated, at least in part, by Dr. T's belief that this might help in dealing with one particularly unreasonable and obstreperous son, Shimon. Although I can now testify from personal experience to the accuracy of Dr. T's assessment of Shimon, it's not clear to me that I was of any help.

The issues raised about prognosis, and the resolution, that the only criterion for treatment decisions should be Mr. L's comfort, were not remarkable. In younger men in a permanent locked-in state, life has been sustained at the hospital for some years, to little purpose that anyone could see. Mr. L could not in any event be heroically maintained for any prolonged period, and the best medical outcome would be the worst personal one: initiation into a stable locked-in life for some shorter period. The resolution: Infections will not be treated and feeding will not be instituted. The breathing tube will remain in (to fend off aspiration) as long as is safe (about two and a half weeks from insertion) and then will be removed; he will not have a tube surgically placed. He will not be resuscitated in the case of a cardiac arrest.

Two issues are worthy of note:

1. Mr. L had prepared a mandate [the local legal mechanism that does the job of a "living will"] in February, assigning Levi to be his mandatary, that is, the person who shall render medical decisions on his father's behalf in the event that his father should become incompetent. The mandate included instructions that in the event of permanent incapacity, heroic life-

prolonging measures are to be avoided, but all comfort measures, including those that will result in reduced lifespan, are to be adopted.

Procedurally, the mandate cannot take effect without legal recognition that the mandate is valid and operative. This process, known as homologation, must be done by a court official, either a superior court judge or a court prothonotary. According to the latest government bulletin dealing with these issues, the *Mot de la Curateur,* homologation currently takes between one and three months (!). Under any circumstance or choice of treatment, this delay represents either some sizable fraction or multiple of Mr. L's expected lifespan, whatever treatment might be provided. It is plausible that Mr. L, or someone like him, in preparing such a document, dreaded most precisely the situation in which he now finds himself (if he is locked in rather than comatose and insensate)—helpless in bed, unable to communicate, the victim of medical perpetrations. This fact of legal life is intolerable. Canadian courts had recently been letting accused child molesters go free because the delay in bringing them to trial represents a violation of their rights, but the law in Quebec intends to let patients languish in hospital because it is unable to come up with a workable approach to homologation.

There was a positive side to this, however: The specific instructions in the mandate, homologated or homogenized or whatever, should not be taken as writ, holy or secular. The mandate had been prepared by a Quebec notary, using some standard form he had lying around the office. All of the children were certain that their father would not have had any input into the drafting and would not have attended to the notary's reading of the thing. He never had any patience for legal documents of any sort; anecdotes were told to this effect, like the time he was buying a household appliance. The salesperson was trying to describe the models and features available, and Mr. L impatiently handed her a blank check and told her to just fill it in with the right amount. In addition, there could have been an issue of his competency at the time of preparing the mandate if it were to be taken seriously. At the time of his stroke in January a fairly obvious memory impairment was noted.

As a matter of fact, the mandatary, Levi, was not going to exercise his powers under it (which, as a matter of fact, would not exist until it was too late), so I spared the family the tale of the mandate. He wanted to go along with the consensus of the family and would not otherwise issue instructions. Until a mandate is in force, this procedure of seeking consensus (if not unanimity) among the nearest relatives, the siblings, would seem to be in accord with the law.

Substantively, there was agreement about the kind of life Mr. L found worth living. He was very active, and still went downhill skiing into his late seventies. He had always said he didn't want nursing home care, and had recently said that if he could no longer drive his car he might as well be dead.

2. The brother Shimon was indeed unbelievably aggravating—not just to the staff and to me but to the other members of his family as well. In fact, I asked Levi afterward whether his brother was married, since I couldn't imagine anybody voluntarily dealing with him on a long-term basis, and Levi said, "Not married, imprisoned! His wife is as bad as he is, and they deserve each other; it's G-d's justice!"

Shimon was the only sibling holding out for aggressive treatment, but he did this in an inconsistent way. At various times he claimed to want a "code" called in the case of a cardiopulmonary arrest, including if necessary a tracheotomy and ventilation, as well as all other measures like antibiotics and gastrostomy (for artificial feeding); at other times, when confronted with what these measures mean and with the prognosis, he said he did not want them. More than once, in fact, he denied ever having said he wanted them.

It would take someone with more psychological knowledge than I possess to explain just why Shimon was so difficult, but a few points stand out:

At least twice, after lengthy explanations of the disease and future course, he would preface his remarks by saying, "We know nothing and we know everything; everything's possible and nothing's possible." He would go on from there to argue for some treatment, in complete and utter disregard of the uselessness of that treatment (if Mr. L is comatose) or its cruelty (if he is or will be locked in), because that was predicated upon understanding what had been said before, which his preamble indicated hadn't occurred. Charitably, we could say that in the context of this medical crisis he was in a state of denial, unable to process information: When asked what he wants to happen, he said, "For my father to dance out of this place." But I don't buy that. From the reactions of his siblings, this was something he did all the time: to seize upon the smallest doubt, uncertainty, ambiguity, or inconsistency in somebody's statement as a reason for totally disregarding the statement (and the person making it).

Several times he would bumptiously say, "We're just wasting time here. So let's get to the bottom line and finish already." If he is sincere about wanting aggressive treatment, then it's hard to see how his arguing with his family who disagree with this, thereby convincing them to sustain his father's life, is wasting time. If the issue is humanely managing a dying process, similar conclusions follow.

Twice, with an air of sage assurance and conclusive and irrefutable wisdom, he said, "So why don't we do what I say, and then we'll have time to argue about it two months later at Dad's bedside." This was said to leave the impression that his was the voice of reasonable temporizing and even compromise. Given what is at stake here, this is roughly equivalent to an argument between someone who wants to execute a condemned prisoner and Torquemada, who would prefer to torture the prisoner as long as he can take it. Torquemada says, "Why don't we do what I say, and we'll have time to argue about it later."

Dr. T speculated that Shimon may have been overcompensating, that he probably had a dreadful relationship with his father. I take it as given that any relationship Shimon has with any sentient being is a dreadful relationship. Dr. T went on to reason that Shimon is trying to redeem this relationship now by acting as his father's "defender." Maybe. Or maybe not. The bottom line is: Not every family member can be reached.

Following a parent's instructions on treatment contained in a living will is a means of fulfilling the duty of reverent obedience, *morah*. But there are limits to *morah* itself: The parent's instructions are not to be obeyed if they conflict with one's obligations to others or to G-d. The source verse itself indicates this: "Each of you shall fear his mother and father, and guard my Sabbaths; I am G-d."[47] Important as parental obedience is, it does not justify violations of the Torah's commandments. And those commandments themselves restrict the autonomy of patients when making medical decisions. *Sefer Chasidim* rules accordingly that a father who asked his son to provide him with food or drink against medical instructions need not be obeyed.[48]

I argue in a later section of this work that Judaism not only allows for but requires persons to exercise judgment in choosing between medical alternatives (Section 2) and, in the final section, that the scope of allowable patient choice grows the closer his or her death approaches (Section 4). The preparation of a living will becomes therefore an exercise in responsible choice on the part of the parent; ensuring that its provisions are fulfilled is a duty of *morah* incumbent upon the patient's children. However, just as most persons die without ever having prepared a will, most patients lapse into incompetence without having prepared a living will. Moreover, as we saw in the case of Mr. L, the circumstances or provisions of a living will may still fail to clarify critical medical choices. One of the most important of those for a child is ensuring that the parent not suffer indignity in the course of a hospitalized dying; it is to that subject that we now turn.

Duties of Children: Preventing Pain and Indignity

In addition to *kibud* and *morah*, placing the child under positive obligations toward the parent, we noted earlier the negative aspects of filial duty: refraining from those actions that cause the parent harm, pain, or indignity. Sadly, the hospital experience of a patient with a terminal illness is likely to seem to include liberal doses of harm, pain, and, most particularly, indignity. A family member who speaks for the voiceless patient by approving or denying medical treatment must inevitably confront the need of deciding when, on balance, the advantages that some treatments offer are outweighed by their associated harms of pain and indignity.

ETHICS CONSULTATION: "SAINT JAMES INFIRMARY"

This case concerned Mrs. C, a sixty-one-year-old woman with a complicated form of Alzheimer's disease with additional physical disability due to frontal impairment of the brain, as well as confirmed multi-infarct dementia [brain damage caused by a series of small strokes]. The course of her disease had begun three years past with tics in the left arm and shoulder, and progressed one year ago to trouble with walking. However, she was living at home with her husband until her hospital admission one month ago. On admission, she had seizures and was found to have low blood glucose levels. Since that time, she has gotten progressively worse despite tests and treatment. Communicative at first, she has become increasingly less oriented and less communicative. At this point in time, her husband claims that she no longer can recognize him. She cannot respond in any meaningful way to questions asked of her.

She was seen in consultation by Dr. D (the hospital's chief of geriatrics) as well, who was unable to attend this meeting. It was confirmed that there is nothing reversible about her condition. She does not have any acute illnesses at this time.

The question raised concerns of continuing nutrition and hydration of this woman. She has needed to be restrained to prevent her from pulling out the intravenous. She has been fairly vigorous at pulling out tubes, including, on at least two occasions, success in pulling out a Foley catheter after the balloon had been inflated. On Monday, her husband brought up the question of feeding, saying that he did not want her to be fed any longer. In his view, he said, "she's not a human being anymore." In addition, to him, "having a life by means of these tubes is not living." Dr. E mentioned that the husband brought up this request after it had become clear that there was nothing reversible in Mrs. C.'s condition. The husband is a Jewish, nonobservant concentration camp survivor.

With nutrition, the current downhill course would be expected to continue. Dr. D estimates that she would survive perhaps another two months on a nourishing regimen. The only safe means of providing her with food would be by surgical insertion of a tube into her stomach, which would require close restraint during a healing period of about ten days.

One would need a heart of stone to fail to sympathize with Mr. C's plight. His wife lies in a hospital. Her mental deterioration has robbed her of even the slim comfort of a familiar face, now that she no longer recognizes her husband. Beyond the reach of pleasure, she is, however, not beyond the reach of pain. The cost of briefly prolonging this sad existence is a surgical procedure to tube-feed her. She would need to be tied down until her surgical incision has healed. Some demented patients become agitated when placed in restraints, struggling against them to the point of exhaustion. If that happens, she will need to be sedated.

Is it relevant to note that Mr. C is a survivor of a Nazi concentration camp? It may be. One of the saddest spectacles of all is to see a demented survivor in restraints, whose shouts reveal that he has confused the current hospitalization with being imprisoned and tormented in a concentration camp. Mrs. C is not herself a survivor, but little imagination is needed to recognize the resonances that restraining his wife may elicit in Mr. C.

Kibud in Its Negative Sense: Preventing Undignified Death

While he did not express it in these terms, Mr. C's plea would likely be construed as a wish that his wife be allowed to die—to meet her inevitable death, shortly to arrive despite anything any doctor or hospital facility may do—with dignity. Yet to say that may be to go too far. His plea may have been the simpler, and more precise, wish that she be spared pain and indignity—shame—in her last moments of living.

Although much has been written about the patient's right to die with dignity, little is offered in the way of describing what a dignified death or dying process is like. This is not in itself surprising. We do not, after all, share any common idea of what constitutes living with dignity; why should we agree about dying with dignity? Perhaps the problem is in presuming that there is one single valued way to die, one "death with dignity."

I want therefore to pursue a smaller and more manageable task, of describing ways in which dying may be made shameful and humiliating. Persons are as a rule more likely to share aversions than preferences, and so it is often easier to describe wrongs, harms, things that we hate about dying, than positive aspects of the process that we all value and wish to experience. Having done that, we need to face the further issue of how Jewish sources might respond to such concerns. At any rate, I believe that Mr. C, and many relatives of the dying, often have quite a clear concept of what is wrong about dying without necessarily having any vision of the ideal death.

The Anatomy of Shame and Humiliation

What is likely to make us see shame and humiliation in a hospital death? Rather than a single answer, I think many different aspects of a patient's experience conspire in this direction. There is, first of all, that shame which is unavoidably connected with any dying; as Schneider writes, "Shame and death are close-linked. The ties are many. Death, along with suffering, deep grief, pain, and violence, belongs to those human experiences that are appropriately veiled from public view. They are deeply vulnerable to shameful public intrusion and profaning violation."[49] Death shames one by making one an object for others to view, by robbing one of one's ability to control how one will be perceived; and dying shames one by leading to death. But that is no more than a sad fact, and it does not distinguish what is specifically felt to be undignified and humiliating about dying in a hospital.

A common focus for that specific shame is the tubes going in and out of a patient. Those tubes going in are for feeding, and those going out are for excretion; this is a truth both about reality and about symbolism, about fact and about perception. Both eating and excretion have been, throughout history and in many different cultures, focal experiences for shame.[50] Being tied to those tubes denies the patient the ability to control the involvement of others in these private activities. The tubes are, moreover, transparent, laying bare the patient's private needs for all to see.

A second and related focus for that shame is helplessness. For many patients, their greatest humiliation occurs when they lose control over excretion, "lying there and being cleaned up like a baby." Many would, and some do, choose death over that embarrassment. But loss of control in itself, without regard to the function in question, is a powerful source of shame; even as retaining control, however it be used, preserves one's dignity. As the rabbis state: "There is no comparison between one who treats himself without dignity, *mitbaze meatzmo,* to one who is treated by another without dignity."[51] Death is of course the ultimate loss of control, and so shameful; but dying in hospital, subject to the intrusions and schedules of others, is not far behind.

Perhaps the ultimate source of shame for a patient in hospital is the exposure that he or she experiences, the uncovering, exemplified but not exhausted by the hospital gown open in back, by the physical examination conducted without closing the door or drawing the curtain. The association between shame and being uncovered is one that reaches well back into history, and it is engrained within the very language we use:

> Our words for shame derive from two Indo-European roots, both with the same meaning. One cluster of words includes our English words custody, hide (both as a noun meaning "skin" and as a verb meaning "conceal"), house, hut, shoe, and sky. In terms of meaning, the common thread in these otherwise disparate words is their relation to covering. In terms of

derivation, each of these words derives from an Indo-European root *(s)que-; *(s)qewa-, which means "to cover." From this same root comes the Lithuanian word kuvetis meaning "to be ashamed." A second Indo-European root *(s)kem-; *(s)kam-, also meaning "to cover," gives us both our English word shame as well as the English camera, the French chemise, and the German Hemd. Shame, then, is intimately linked to the need to cover—in particular, to cover that which is exposed.[52]

Behind the literal truth, that "shame" derives from "uncovered," stands an even more important recognition of their symbolic connection. The Talmud describes a conversation R Ze'ira had with R Yehuda when he saw the latter was in a playful mood [chazya d'have b'dicha da'atei]. R Ze'ira asked why garments are called by the term l'vusha. R Yehuda responded that the source of the word l'vusha is lo bush: no shame.[53]

The Prohibition Against Allowing an Undignified Death: Kibud, Morah, and Causing Pain

These are some of the main elements contributing indignity to a dying process. From a Jewish point of view, I believe, they must be considered by the adult child who is responsible for arranging the appropriate care for a parent. To neglect them certainly represents a failure to satisfy the positive commandment of respectful service, kibud. In addition, if the parent has prepared a living will that deals with these matters, the failure to implement these instructions is a violation of reverent obedience, morah. Such neglect is even more serious than the failure to fulfill these positive commandments, however, because I believe that it represents a violation of the scriptural prohibitions against striking or cursing a parent.[54]

These two prohibitions implicate a general obligation to avoid causing pain or shame to the parent. To the extent that the patient's child is capable of directing or influencing the way in which treatment will be provided, the child is culpable for the avoidable pain or shame incurred by that patient.[55]

A theoretical distinction helps to clarify and strengthen the point. The first verse, prohibiting striking a parent,[56] prohibits causing pain; in general, Jewish tradition treats psychological pain—anguish—at least as seriously as it does physical pain. A good example of this is found in *Sefer Chasidim*,[57] dealing with the case of a son who, in an attempt to spare his parents pain, threatens them that he will initiate a fast unless they agree not to fast themselves. This is prohibited, the author writes, "since his father and mother have more pain from his fast than from their own."

The Prohibition Against Allowing an Undignified Death: *Bizayon* [Humiliation]

I have said that the second verse,[58] which prohibits a child from cursing his parents, also prohibits his causing them indignity, shame, or humiliation.[59] The connection between these two may seem obscure. In fact, the concept of cursing and that of indignity are etymologically identical in Hebrew. The term for cursing, whose root is *KLL,* is a verbal form deriving from *KL. KL* itself means, literally, "light" in the sense of "lacking in weight." To *KLL* someone therefore means to treat that person "lightly," without dignity. "To curse," *KLL,* therefore, is, in Hebrew, the precise linguistic and conceptual antonym to the act of "honoring," *KBD,* the same term found in the Fifth Commandment, which, as we had seen, means literally to treat the parents in a "weighty" manner.[60]

For most practical purposes, either derivation will serve the same purpose.[61] There is one potential difference between them, however, which looms large in our context. I have argued that the adult child's responsibility to care for an incompetent parent requires close attention to shame and indignity. It is, however, often true in these cases that the patient is, or seems to be, oblivious to social aspects of treatment, for example, of being disrobed. If the parent is unaware of being treated in a shameful or undignified way, has the child violated his responsibility by allowing such treatment? Or, as the staff of a geriatric unit will sometimes argue, does his scrupulousness under these circumstances indicate that he is more concerned about his own perception of the proprieties than about his obligation to his parents?

To respond to these questions, it is necessary to distinguish between anguish and shame or indignity. The patient's own perceptions are the only possible measure of anguish or any other forms of pain. What a person cannot feel cannot pain him. Because the anguish associated with the experience of shame requires a considerable degree of self-awareness and abstract thought, patients with brain damage may well lose the capacity for that form of social pain we call shame before they lose the capacity to experience physical pain. I take this to express a logical truth about the concept "I was in pain, but felt nothing"; if meant literally, it is a logical contradiction.

But indignity, and its associated harm, is different. A person need not be aware of having been humiliated to be in fact humiliated; and a person need not experience the harm of being shamed in order to be shamed. Unlike pain, therefore, which is a truth about the patient's own perceptions, humiliation (in Hebrew, *bizayon*) at least incorporates (without necessarily being restricted to) a truth about the perceptions others have of the patient. A deeply demented patient who is left bare before the sight of every hospital passer-by feels no pain at this fact, but the person who that patient is has nonetheless been shamed by it. The child who is that parent's caretaker but fails to address this indignity has not violated the prohibition against causing the parent pain, but has violated the injunction against "cursing" the parent, that is, treating the parent "lightly."

Pain and Shame as Legal Categories in Treating the Dying Parent

What, then, is the measure of shame, if not solely the person's own reaction to treatment, and what is its connection, if any, to pain? Several sources can be brought to bear:

1. It is clear that a child is required to formally demonstrate honor of the parent even following the parent's death, despite the fact that the parent is (from the mundane point of view) insensible of that fact. By strict logic, it follows that a child is required to refrain from humiliating a parent even if the par-

ent is unaware of the act.[62] As the Jewish mystical classic the *Zohar* says,

> "Honor your father and your mother": This *mitzva* obligates him [the child] during life; after their death, should we say perhaps that he is free of it? It is not so, for even after death he is obligated to honor them, and even more so than during their lifetimes.[63]

2. The voluntary reaction of the competent parent toward a child's actions determines whether that action constitutes honor or humiliation; or, in other words, behavior that would be considered insulting by one parent is accepted, or even valued, by another. A good example of this principle, which has been accepted as authoritative law,[64] is supplied when the mother of R Yishmael claims the "honor" of washing the feet of her son.[65]

3. The reaction of a parent can, however, only be conclusive in its effect if that person is in full possession of his or her faculties. On behalf of incompetent persons, the measure of humiliation depends upon an estimation of how a member of that person's group would ordinarily react to the situation at hand. For example: In general, the guardian of the estate of orphans who are incompetent (e.g., because they are minors) is not permitted to use their funds for charity.[66] An exception to that rule: If the father of the orphans had provided financially for impoverished relatives, the guardian may continue these charitable disbursements. Failure to continue these provisions, to satisfy this familial duty, is considered a cause of shame to both the (deceased) father and to the orphans, both of whom are objectively shamed by this failure to carry out a familial duty.[67]

4. A similar point emerges from an important source in the Talmud that deals with shame and pain in the context of the court's carrying out a legal execution.[68] There is a rabbinic disagreement over whether men dread physical pain more than

they do humiliation, but common ground that the shame of being naked in public is more grievous for women than for men.[69] Here too, therefore, the law determines the fact of indignity on the basis of the normal reaction of an average member of the category in question.

No easy resolution of the dilemmas of caring for an incompetent patient will necessarily emerge from these sources. For one thing, the obligations may work at cross purposes: Sparing a parent pain may cause indignity; service may conflict with obedience.[70] Patients do not come neatly tagged as "competent" or "incompetent," judgments made particularly difficult in the hospital context, with the confounding factors of illness and a patient's reactions to treatment. The difficulty of defining competence, which will be dealt with at length in Section 3, emerges in an interesting way from the case just considered. Why not simply ask the prisoner for his or her preference when leaving for the execution? The earlier principle, that a competent person's reaction to treatment is definitive of what shall count as "honor" or "indignity," suggests this obvious solution. The key may well lie in questioning the presumption that the prisoner could competently respond. As a matter of fact, those taken out to execution were drugged to blunt their pain;[71] under the influence of this mind-altering medication, they may be judged no longer capable of expressing a competent choice.

Difficult as they are, it may be argued that judgments of competency are matters requiring legal or medical expertise, restricting the family's role to providing input. Once a patient has been designated as incompetent, a whole series of new and difficult questions arises: interpreting and applying prior directives, weighing of pain and indignity against medical benefits, and so on. In some cases, it is clear to everyone that a patient should continue to be treated aggressively; sometimes, it is equally clear that a patient's comfort rather than cure should be the prime consideration. But oftentimes, these questions leave the case in a "gray area"; reasonable people will disagree over what kind of treatment is most appropriate. And the question now is: Whose judgment in the gray area should control?

The Priority of Duty

To clarify this question of "Who shall decide?" we need to recall the contrast explored earlier in this section between the "standard view" about family involvement and the duty perspective that emerges from the Jewish sources that have been examined.

The Regimes of Right and of Duty: Procedural Implications

In the standard view, as we saw, there is no need to involve the family in medical decision making when there exists a satisfactory alternative. Although the family in that view has a defeasible right to decide, this right is based upon their knowledge of and respect for the patient's interests and preferences. When those abilities are claimed to be better served by another mechanism—doctor, hospital ethics committee, or judge—the only question is whether the claim is credible; if it is, there is no reason in logic, law, or ethics for the family's role to be preserved. For that reason, perhaps, the concern for potential family conflict of interest is given so much emphasis in the standard view. Any plausible allegation of conflict may as well be accepted, since there is no moral cost associated with using a decision maker external to the family.

For the standard view, then, the family's involvement is, under defined circumstances, strictly dispensable. Recall the case of Mrs. A, the long-term psychiatric patient whose existence had been concealed from her daughter. The issue was whether a niece should continue to make decisions regarding Mrs. A's medical care or whether the daughter should now be contacted. The hospital and its consulting ethicist, under the sway of the standard view, ruled in favor of the niece (and of continuing concealment from the daughter that her mother yet lives and wishes to see her).

This conclusion is unacceptable from the point of view of duty—and its consequences, in the case of Mrs. A's daughter, are utterly repugnant. The duty perspective insists that the right thing be done, and done in the right way, by or with the involvement of the right person.

Someone else can feed or clothe my parent, true; and, often enough, I am constrained to rely upon another to perform the physical action. (A son or daughter must rely upon the medical staff to insert a feeding tube, for example.) As long as that other person is acting on my behalf, as my agent, I may be said to be fulfilling my filial duty to my parent, but not otherwise. The protection of the patient is, of course, paramount, and if a family is neglectful of or fundamentally mishandling its responsibilities, then naturally an outside decision maker must be invoked. That contingency must be avoided in any reasonable manner consistent with the patient's safety, however, for from the perspective of duty, it is essential that through medical decisions, as through many other acts, the children be enabled to fulfill their filial obligation.

Family Decision Making in the "Gray Zone"

Medical decision making for incompetent patients is replete with decisions about which reasonable people disagree, ethical dilemmas so finely balanced that no fully persuasive argument on either side is in prospect. These decisions may concern treatments of uncertain benefit and indeterminate harm, in short, medical gambling—so that the decision maker's reaction is forced to rely upon how he or she feels about rolling the dice (see Section 4). In other cases, while the results are relatively certain, how to value those results is up for dispute: The only way to nourish Mrs. C is by surgically inserting a feeding tube into her stomach, but she will then need to be physically restrained from tugging at the tube and perhaps "chemically restrained" with tranquilizers as well. Is the gain worth the loss? In yet other cases, although the patient had, while competent, provided advance instruction, the directive yields in the present circumstances no clear guidance.

Many other such instances can be provided; such insoluble dilemmas are the heart, for better or worse, of the bioethics literature. At the end of the day, no convincing arguments have been found, and yet a decision must be made. The question is: Who shall make that decision? Whose moral judgment will hold sway within the gray zone? To sharpen the issue, let us assume that the patient's son and the patient's physician are in strong disagreement, for the fact that a dispute yields to no definitive conclusion does not necessarily leave the disputants amicably "agreeing to disagree."

In such cases, failing any convincing argument on either side, the perspective of duty entails that the family's strong feelings should be granted precedence.[72] For both doctor and son, it is true, the care of the patient involves duty's demands; and I would not hold professional duty in any lower regard than filial obligation. But the doctor has many other patients, while the son and daughter have only the one father. Should the decision of the children violate the physician's conscience, the doctor's recourse is clear: He may remove himself from the case. (And, should no other doctor be prepared to follow the son's decision, we have strong grounds to suspect our premise was false: This dispute does not involve a clash between two reasonable positions.)

The Claims of Strict Obligation

Put in Jewish terms, while the doctor performs a *mitzva* in treating the patient, the claim of the children to determine the course of medical treatment is one of strict obligation *[chovah]*. In cases of a clash between the demands of a *mitzva* and *chovah*, priority is given to *chovah*.[73]

A good example of the priority of duty is found in a responsum of the eighteenth-century Italian R Chayim Yosef David 'Azula'i (popularly known by his acronym, Chida).[74] The issue: Re'uven's wife is about to give birth and nobody in town is a *mohel* (one who performs circumcision). A man has come to Re'uven and said, "Don't worry. You don't know, after all, whether your wife will give birth to a boy; and even if she does, I am prepared to perform the circumcision myself. Even though I have never performed a circumcision before," he "reassured" the father, "I am quite confident that I can do this. Moreover," this man added, "if you refuse to give your son over to me for the performance of the circumcision, the community can force you to do this, as it has the power to force you to obey the commandments." The father wanted to know whether this man is right or whether he is permitted to delay the circumcision beyond its usual time limit to allow a competent *mohel* to arrive at the town.

Chida reassures Re'uven that he is within his rights to resist this offer, on grounds that the "medical treatment" proposed, circumcision, is risky in his "friend's" untried hands. He quotes Rambam,[75] who had ruled that "the son of a man is not circumcised without that man's knowledge or consent"—*da'at,* a term of interesting ambiguity for our purposes. Moreover, as Chida notes, this principle was generalized in a commentary on Rambam written by R Yosef Karo, who also authored the authoritative code of Jewish law, *Shulchan Arukh.* R Yosef Karo explains Rambam's general principle to be "When a commandment is incumbent upon one person another may not perform it without the first person's knowledge."[76]

Several aspects of the case of circumcision are suggestive for our purposes.

1. The father labors under a strict obligation—*chovah*—to circumcise the son.

2. Most fathers do not have the expertise of the *mohel.* Therefore, the usual manner in which the father discharges this obligation is by appointing a *mohel* his agent for this purpose. Since the *mohel* acts with the father's authority and at his direction, the father is legally considered to have satisfied his personal obligation.

3. The circumcision generally may not be performed without the father's knowledge and consent, and one who usurps the father's prerogative has wronged him, even if the circumcision is competently performed.[77]

4. This case poses a moral dilemma over the manner in which the circumcision of Re'uven's son should be performed. None of the alternative choices is ideal: Either the safety of the act will be compromised, or its timely performance will be sacrificed. Since the strict obligation, *chovah,* rests upon the father, it is the father's task to weigh these factors and decide upon a resolution.

5. The entire community is under a more general obligation to see to it that children are circumcised. If the father fails to fulfill his own obligation in a reasonable way, the court is charged to step in and to see to it that the circumcision is performed.[78]

The same can be said, point for point, regarding the moral role of adult children in determining how an incompetent parent should be treated from the point of view of a regime of duty:

1. Children labor under strict obligations to care for their parents: the obligation of *kibud,* dutiful service; of *morah,* reverent obedience; and the strict injunctions to avoid causing their parents pain and shame.
2. Most children do not have the expertise required to perform the medical acts required by these obligations. Therefore, the usual manner in which children discharge this obligation is by appointing experts to act as their agents in providing medical care.
3. It is the prerogative of the children to fulfill their obligations by participating in these medical decisions. One who usurps this role, even when providing competent and appropriate medical care, has wronged them.
4. Some cases of medical care pose moral dilemmas; none of the treatment alternatives is ideal. In such cases, because the role of the children in medical decision making is one of strict obligation, their weighting of the relevant factors and judgment should ordinarily be conclusive.[79]
5. The community, however, retains a general obligation to ensure that incompetent patients are not medically harmed or neglected. When the decisions of children are clearly wrong, the court is obliged to step in and order that appropriate care be provided.

Endnotes

1. Elaine B. Krasik, "Comment: The Role of the Family in Medical Decisionmaking for Incompetent Adult Patients: A Historical Perspective and Case Analysis," *University of Pittsburgh Law Review* 48 (1987): 539, at 541 (emphases added).
2. Allen Buchanan and Dan Brock, *Deciding for Others* (New York:

Cambridge University Press, 1989): 136; see also Nancy Rhoden, "Litigating Life and Death," *Harvard Law Review* 102 (1988): 375–446.*

3. Buchanan and Brock (1989).*

4. Buchanan and Brock (1989).*

5. Buchanan and Brock (1989); compare with Krasik (1987): 555–557.*

6. Benjamin Freedman, "On the Rights of the Voiceless," *The Journal of Medicine and Philosophy* 3 (1978): 196–210.*

7. Buchanan and Brock (1988): 142 ff.

8. *In re* West, 212 N.Y.S. 2d 832 (1961), at 834.

9. See Krasik (1987): 554.

10. *In re* Spring, 380 Mass. 629, 405 N. E. 2d 115, 122 n. 3 (1980).

11. *In re* Guardianship of Roe, 383 Mass. 415, 421 N.E. 2d 40, 56 (1981).

12. *In re* Conroy, 98 N.J. 321, 486 A.2d 1209, 1218 (1985).

13. Krasik (1987): 550.

14. Jonathan Moreno, "Who's to Choose? Surrogate Decisionmaking in New York State," *Hastings Center Report* 23, no. 1 (1993): 5–11, at 8.

15. Karl Popper, *The Logic of Scientific Discovery* (Toronto: University of Toronto Press, 1959).

16. Compare with *Foody v. Manchester Memorial Hospital*, 40 Conn. Supp. 127, 482 A.2d 713, 717 (1984).

17. *Ritz v. Florida Patient's Compensation Fund*, 436 So. 2d 987 (Fla. Dist. Ct. App. 1983).

18. John Hardwig, "What About the Family?" *Hastings Center Report* 20, no. 2 (1990): 5–10 (emphases in original). Compare with Patricia A. King, "The Authority of Families to Make Medical Decisions for Incompetent Patients After the Cruzan Decision," *Journal of Law, Medicine and Health Care* 19 (1991): 76–79; and James Lindemann Nelson, "Taking Families Seriously," *Hastings Center Report* 22, no. 4 (1992): 6–12.*

19. See Ronald J. Christie and C. Barry Hoffmaster, *Ethical Issues in Family Medicine* (New York: Oxford University Press, 1986); and many articles by Ian McWhinney.

20. Hardwig (1990): 8.

21. See Melinda Friend and Jochen Vollmann, "Case Study: For Love or

Money," *Hastings Center Report* 25, no. 4 (1995): 22–23.

22. Linda and Ezekiel Emanuel, "Decisions at the End of Life: Guided by Communities of Patients," *Hastings Center Report* 23, no. 5 (1993): 7.

23. A. B. Seckler, D. E. Meier, M. Mulvihill, and B. E. Cammer Paris, "Substituted Judgment: How Accurate Are Proxy Predictions?" *Annals of Internal Medicine* 115 (1991): 92–98, at 95.

24. Since writing this section, a newspaper account of a situation similar in many respects appeared: David Foster, "Son Reunited with Mother He Thought Was Dead," *Montreal Gazette,* May 14 (1995): A1.*

25. Joanne Lynn, "Why I Don't Have a Living Will," *Journal of Law, Medicine and Health Care* 19 (1991): 101–104, at 103.

26. Dallas High, "All in the Family: Extended Autonomy and Expectations in Surrogate Health Care Decision-Making," *The Gerontologist* 28 Supp. (1988): 46–51.

27. Ps. 119.162.

28. George Fletcher, *Loyalty* (New York: Oxford University Press, 1993): 86.

29. Decisions of the Israeli Rabbinic Court, A, no. 145 (emphasis added).

30. See Robert Cover, "Obligation: A Jewish Jurisprudence of the Social Order," *Journal of Law and Religion* 5 (1988): 65–74, at 67.*

31. Lev. 19.3.

32. Ex. 21.15, 21.17.

33. Ex. 20.12.

34. TB *Kidushin* 31b.

35. Cover (1988): 71.

36. See Rambam, *Peirush Hamishnayot* TB *Kidushin* 29a.*

37. Contrast with Responsa *Michtam leDavid Yore Dei'a,* section 33.*

38. Compare with *Torat Kohanim* Lev. 19.3.*

39. Rambam, *Mishne Tora, Hilkhot Mamrim,* 6.10.

40. *Shulchan Arukh Yore Dei'a* 240.10.

41. Gerald Blidstein, *Honor Thy Father and Mother* (New York: Ktav Publishing, 1975): 118.

42. Rambam, *Mishne Tora, Hilkhot Gerushin* 10.23.

43. Responsa *Tzitz Eli'ezer,* vol. 12, section 59.

44. A stance he attributes to *D'risha, Tur, Yore Dei'a* 240 note 2.

45. Based in part upon Radvaz's commentary on Rambam, *Hilkhot Mamrim* 6.10.

46. R. J. Moss and J. LaPuma, "The Ethics of Medical Restraints" *Hastings Center Report* 21, no. 1 (1991): 22–25.

47. Lev. 19.3.

48. *Sefer Chasidim* 234; see also *Sefer Kibud Av V'em*, R Ya'akov Pinchas Feldman privately printed, Jerusalem (1990): 17.*

49. Carl D. Schneider, *Shame, Exposure and Privacy* (Boston: Beacon Press, 1977): 77.*

50. See Schneider (1977), Chapter 7; compare with TB *P'sachim* 82.*

51. TY *Taanit* 2.

52. Schneider (1977): 29–30.

53. TB *Shabbat* 77b.

54. Ex. 21.15 and 21.17.

55. Responsa *Meishiv Davar,* part 2, section 50.

56. Ex. 21.15.

57. *Sefer Chasidim,* section 340.

58. Ex. 21.17.

59. See *Sefer Hachinuch* 260.*

60. Compare with Deut. 27.16.*

61. For that reason the responsa literature often treats psychological pain and humiliation in common. See, for example, Responsa *Zichron Yehuda,* sec. 78, s.v. *ken ira*; see also R Moshe Feinstein, *Igrot Moshe, Yore Dei'a,* vol. 2, section 63, s.v. *al kol panim kevan.**

62. Responsa R Akiva Eiger, section 68, s.v. *vhine baguf.**

63. Zohar, *B'chukotai* 115b.

64. R Tzvi Hershel Schechter, "Regarding Laws of Death and a 'Dead Man'" *(B'dinei meit v'gavra k'tila),* in R Mordechai Halperin, ed., *Sefer Assia,* vol. 7 (Jerusalem: Falk-Schlesinger Institute, 1993): 188–206, at 203, who quotes Responsa Maharam Schick (*Yore Dei'a,* section 218).

65. Compare with *Tzitz Eli'ezer,* part 7, section 49, *Kuntres Even Ya'akov;* Responsa *Yabia Omer,* part 5, *Yore Dei'a,* section 21; and Responsa *Meishiv Davar,* part 2, section 50.*

66. TB *Gitin,* chapter *Hanizakin.*

67. See Responsa Mahari Mintz, 1, s.v. *nir'e li;* compare Responsa Ya'avetz, vol. 1, section 2, s.v. *v'khatav hod.**

68. See TB *Sanhedrin* 44b–45a.*

69. See TY *K'tubot* 5.8 and TB *K'tubot* 67.*

70. I am grateful to Professor Karen Lebacqz for this point.*

71. See TB *Sanhedrin* 43a.

72. For a striking responsum on this, see R Moshe Feinstein, Responsa *Igrot Moshe Choshen Mishpat* 2, section 74.*

73. See Responsa *Radvaz* 3, section 208, and R Shabtai Rapaport, "Priorities in Allocating Public Funds for Medicine" (in Hebrew), in R Mordechai Halperin, ed., *Sefer Assia,* vol. 7 (Jerusalem: Falk-Schlesinger Institute, 1993): 94–106.*

74. Responsa *Chayim Sha'al* 1, number 58.

75. Mishne Torah, *Hilkhot Milah,* chapter 1.

76. *Kesef Mishne,* ibid.

77. See R Naftali Tzvi Yehudah Berlin (N'tziv), Responsa *Meishiv Davar* 3, section 14.

78. Mishne Torah, *Hilkhot Milah,* Chapter 1.

79. See R Moshe Feinstein, Responsa *Igrot Moshe, Choshen Mishpat* 2, section 74; and my discussion in Section 4: Risk.

CONSENT

"the reasonable caretaker" and the obligation to consent

Introduction

Commandment 546: To Build a Fence Around Your Roof

[We are commanded] to remove obstacles and stumbling-blocks from all of our homes; of this was it written, "You shall build a fence around your roof.". . . . For the Holy One graced the bodies of persons by blowing into them a living spirit, intelligence, to guard the body from all harm. . . . And many matters were prohibited by the Sages of blessed memory so that people will be guarded against evil occurrences and harm, for it is inappropriate for an intelligent person to endanger himself. . . . And [this commandment] applies everywhere and at all times, amongst men and women.[1]

Up until this point, we have been considering bioethics from the point of view of a Jewish model of duty owed between persons: health care professionals, patients, and family members. But the Jewish model of duty encompasses a further dimension: duties that one owes regarding oneself, in particular, a duty to protect one's own health through seeking out and undergoing appropriate medical care.

Consent and Duty to the Self

In many ways, this may strike a modern reader as a foreign, obscure, and dangerous concept. How can you "owe" something to yourself, and if you did, why could you not "absolve" yourself of this "obligation"? How could self-regarding obligations be enforced, and by whom? If not enforceable, in what meaningful sense could they still be called duties? What is the content of these obligations? What do they call upon us to do?

Bioethics especially, in its current state, which identifies ethics *tout court* with social ethics, has difficulty accommodating the idea of duties regarding self. The heart of bioethics is the principle of free and informed consent, the right of every competent person to decide about proposed medical treatments after receiving the information that person finds necessary. Discussions of the principle and ramifications of informed consent have in themselves accounted for a substantial proportion of the contemporary literature on bioethics and medical jurisprudence. In addition, the concept always looms large and often dominates the current understanding of physician-patient relationships, as well as the ethical conduct of biomedical research. Although relatively new, the notion of informed consent has come to shape our response to far older bioethical issues as well. For example, the promise of medical confidentiality, a bioethical principle as old as the Hippocratic Oath, is now commonly tempered by informed consent: Medical secrets need not be kept if their potential disclosure was mentioned to and approved by the patient prior to the medical encounter. The moral analysis of new medical interventions and technologies in such areas as reproduction, genetics, and transplantation almost always begins (and not uncommonly ends) with an exploration of how the doctrine of informed consent applies in these new circumstances.

Informed consent is understood to be an expression of untrammeled individual freedom, and duties regarding the self seem to stand in direct contradiction to that principle. Seemingly, one or the other must yield. But the cost of choosing between these two is considerable.

On the one hand, those who embrace consent, in jettisoning self-regarding duties, seem unable to find space for any moral commitment higher than that owed to the individual patient's current act of will. The reason is that the self-regarding duty to responsibly care for one's own health does not simply implicate a bare "duty to self," as may be shown by exposing that concept's equivocation. A self-regarding duty may be defined as such because of the source of the duty, or because of its object. It may, that is, be self-regarding because the duty to act is grounded in one's obligation to oneself (self-regarding duty as source), or because what the duty requires one to do is an action that is directed toward the self, the same person is duty-bound to perform the action (self-regarding duty as object).

Judaism supports self-regarding duties in the second sense. The ultimate source of all obligation, including duties to the self, is to be found not within the self, but through a covenant with G-d. That covenant requires persons to care for their own health, as for that of others (duty as object). But it is this latter meaning that is in most clear contradiction to the current view of informed consent, which sees consent as a mechanism for extending unfettered self-regarding decisions. That is, if informed consent means that one has the right to decide about medical care as one chooses, it is in conflict with a view that one is duty-bound to act toward the self in certain ways—in self-regarding duties as object.

Stewardship and Consent

Judaism is not alone in facing this normative conflict with the ideal of informed consent. Self-regarding duty in this sense, the duty to make prudent choices that express care for one's own health, may derive from any one of a number of sources: obligations to those who rely upon you or care about your well-being; a belief that one's body is to some degree held in trust or stewardship, whether this be on behalf of G-d, some ideal that you hold, or some special mission that is yours to accomplish; duty to your community, or tribe, or any entity larger than yourself. In Roman Catholic thought, for example, duties to self are expressed through restrictions upon allowable surgical procedures, judged by such moral guidelines as the principle of totality.[2] A decision to discard the very possibility of such commitments in the name of informed consent should not be taken lightly.

On the other hand, informed consent is so central to current bioethical discussion that the decision to discard it is also very costly. A duty perspective with no space for consent has no common language with current bioethical study and cannot benefit from any moral insight that those discussions may yield.

These are very sharp horns of a very large dilemma. As stated, there is no reconciling the two sides. I shall therefore try to change the terms of discussion by questioning the received interpretations of both. I shall try to show how an authentic Jewish approach not only permits but also requires persons to intelligently choose how to live their lives, and I shall argue that some main tenets of the doctrine of informed consent may be understood precisely in those terms. This discussion therefore argues on behalf of a new perspective on both consent and Judaism in their relation to health care.

In this section, then, I shall propose one resolution, by an extended exploration of the role consent may play on behalf of one who considers his or her own body to be held in trust. This is a view found in traditional Jewish sources in a firm, unyielding way; it is to those sources that my analysis is directed. I believe, however, that if a Jewish accommodation of consent can be described, then similar tactics could be employed to carve out space for consent within other ethical theories and religious systems that acknowledge self-regarding duties.

The Duty to Seek Medical Treatment

It is common currency among today's writers on Judaism and bioethics that persons are obliged to seek out and accept appropriate medical care and that health care practitioners fulfill a religious commandment by providing such care. (Health care practitioners are almost always, in this literature, understood to be doctors—an anachronistic convention that I will respect in this and the following sections for ease of reference.)

This normative consensus was not reached without opposition. The Bible speaks of numerous miraculous cures effected through prayer and the intervention of prophets.[3] (Here and throughout this work, by "the Bible" I mean solely the works taken into the Jewish scriptural canon.) It does not, however, record any instances of persons being healed by physicians. To the contrary: G-d promises that those who faithfully obey His commandments will be spared all of the illnesses that were visited upon the Egyptians.[4] In the one instance in which the Bible tells us of a patient who sought medical care, namely, Asa, King of Judah, he is criticized for "not pursuing G-d, but [rather] the physicians."[5] Asa promptly died.

Accordingly, there was some medieval resistance to this consensus. Ibn Ezra was of the view that persons may only seek medical assistance for man-made wounds, not for disease or internal afflictions (the latter, presumably, having been Divinely inflicted).[6] His view did not prevail, nor did that of Ramban (Nahmanides), who, while not prohibiting recourse to medicine (see later in this section), felt that it reflects a lack of piety and faith: Ideally, the sick would need no physician other than G-d.[7]

Seeking Healing as a Religious Duty: Proposed Biblical Sources

What is the source of the obligation to heal, and to seek healing? The biblical verse that convinced Ibn Ezra that medical treatment for wounds is permissible describes the payment of damages owed to an assault victim: "He [the assaulter] shall pay for his [the victim's] rest, and shall cause him to be healed." The last clause, *v'rapo y'rapei,* is a grammatically unusual construction; among its possible meanings, and the one most appropriate to this context, is "and shall pay for his healing."[8] The Talmud states of this verse, "From here [we learn] that permission is given to the physician to heal."[9]

Several logically distinct steps are present: If the assaulter is compelled to pay his victim's medical expenses, it follows that

a. a patient is permitted to seek medical attention,
b. a physician is permitted to provide it, and
c. the physician is permitted to charge for his services.

The logical progression is noteworthy because here, as in other Jewish sources, the moral stance of one party (the patient's freedom to seek treatment) is implied through the moral stance of another (the doctor's freedom to charge, or the assailant's duty to pay medical fees). For example: R Isaac Arama, the medieval author of the Bible commentary *Akedat Yitzchak,* notes that since all agree that a physician is permitted to treat patients, it is morally necessary that patients be allowed to seek treatment. Otherwise, by practicing their trade, physicians would violate the injunction against tempting others to do wrong, a prohibition understood by the rabbis as one underlying meaning of the verse "do not place a stumbling block before the blind."[10] But neither the verse in Exodus commanding an assailant to pay his victim's medical fees nor its rabbinic interpretation implies that there exists any *obligation* to seek healing (for the patient) or to heal (for the physician).

Another source, sometimes alleged to establish a duty to seek to be healed, is also in fact permissive in effect. The Bible asserts, "And you shall guard my commandments and perform my statutes, that a person shall do and live with them."[11] On the basis of this verse, a rabbinic conclave established that the protection of life supersedes the obligation to obey Jewish law, with three exceptions (murder, idolatry, and prohibited sexual relations).[12] Despite one author's inference that this may serve to ground an obligation to seek healing,[13] this provision again seems permissive rather than obligatory: In pursuit of healing one is freed from other conflicting obligations.

Seeking Healing as a Religious Duty: Rabbinic Reasoning

There is in fact no biblical verse that clearly asserts an obligation to seek medical attention. However, two verses are commonly pressed into service as requiring that a person take care to guard his own life; from that general injunction, the inference is made that medical care may be one such required measure. The verses are:

> Just take care [hishameir] for yourself, and take great care of your soul, lest you forget these things that your eyes have seen, and lest they shall depart from your heart all the days of your life; and you shall make them known to your children and your children's children.[14]

> And you shall take great care of your souls; for you have not seen any image in the day G-d your Lord spoke to you on Horeb from the midst of fire.[15]

That these verses imply an obligation for a person to take those steps necessary to protect his or her own life is first stated in a talmudic tale:

> Our rabbis learned: It happened that a certain pious man [chasid] was praying at the roadside and a certain nobleman came, and greeted him, and he did not return the greeting. After he had concluded his prayer he [the nobleman] said to him, "Is it not written in your Torah 'Just take care for yourself, and take care of your soul'; and, 'And you shall take great care of your souls'? Why did you not return my greeting?—Were I to

cut off your head with my sword who would exact your blood from my hand!?" He said to him: "Were you standing before a king of flesh and blood, and your friend came and greeted you, would you return the greeting?" He replied, "No." He said, "Considering it is so before a king of flesh and blood, how much more so for me, who was standing before the King of Kings, the Holy One Blessed Be He?" Immediately the official absolved him [*hitpayes;* was conciliated].[16]

In Hebrew idiom, the term "soul" can refer to "life"; thus, it is possible for an expression like "take care of your soul" to mean "take care to protect your life."[17] The interpretation is nonetheless forced, as is noted by one leading talmudic commentator.[18] It is clear from the context of the verses invoked that the primary literal meaning of both verses refers to theological commandments: first, to never forget the commands of the Torah, and second, to guard against thinking of G-d in terms of physical imagery.[19] None of the major Jewish biblical commentators takes either verse as including or intending an injunction to protect one's own life. And it is rare[20] for novel biblical interpretations proposed by impatient Roman noblemen to be accepted by the rabbis.[21] Nevertheless, Rambam codifies the spirit of this interpretation:

> It is a positive commandment to remove every obstacle that presents a danger and to take exceeding care on this matter, as it says, "take care [*hishameir*] for yourself, and take great care of your soul."[22]

In another talmudic passage, the first of these verses is, only somewhat less implausibly, taken to prohibit an act of self-aggression; again, Rambam codifies the law together with its basis in biblical interpretation:

> We learned, one who curses himself transgresses a prohibition, as it says, "take care [*hishameir*] for yourself, and take great care of your soul."[23]

> One who curses himself is corporally punished [i.e., lashed] as
> one who curses others, as it says, "take care *[hishameir]* for
> yourself, and take care of your soul."[24]

(On the true Hebrew meaning of "cursing," see Section 1.)

Another possible biblical source is found in TB *Bava Kamma* 91b,
which states, "A person is forbidden to wound himself, as it is written,
'Yet your blood of your soul shall I require of you.'"[25] Once again, however, the interpretation is forced: In context, this last verse speaks of
murder, rather than suicide; killing, rather than endangering; and actively harming, rather than passively failing to seek medical assistance.

Seeking Healing as a Religious Duty: Implications of Sources and Reasoning

The fact remains that, despite scanty biblical warrant, a clear
norm was established in Judaism that persons are obliged to preserve
and protect their lives, to seek to be healed, if necessary. Given these
derivations, some possible inferences are noteworthy:

- The obligation to seek healing is not a unique injunction,
  is not *sui generis*. It is, rather, continuous with duties regarding other activities of life. As, for example, one is prohibited to travel in dangerous territory (without great
  need) and forbidden to omit the niceties when greeted by
  an irascible nobleman bearing a sword, one is required to
  seek a physician's assistance when ill.
- This duty to live safely is one held in common within the
  community as well. The last-noted derivation claims a
  continuity between murdering another and murdering the
  self. The injunction against cursing oneself is explicitly
  understood by Rambam as identical with the prohibition
  against cursing others. Within a community governed by
  common caring, the self is no less an object of care than is
  the other; within a community of duty, duties to self are
  not distinct in kind from duties to other.
- The duty to protect one's health is relatively insensitive to

the distinction between acts that endanger the self and omissions that result in the same end; perhaps better expressed, the duty serves as the underlying reason for prohibiting those actions that are injurious (e.g., wounding or cursing the self) as well as for requiring those actions that are beneficent (e.g., seeking needed medical attention).

- This duty appears to need no strong biblical warrant, but, at most, a vague allusion. Even a bloodthirsty Roman recognizes the strength of the injunction. The duty of self-protection rather emerges as a rule of reason, as is evident in the talmudic statement "One who is in pain goes to a doctor's office."[26] This statement, cited by some as a normative basis for the duty to seek health care,[27] appears quite differently when understood in context. The Talmud had cited a biblical verse as a proof text serving to establish the procedural principle that one who seeks a court judgment awarding him property that is in the hands of another must bring proof that the property is his. R Ashi questions the very need for a proof text by saying, "This may be learned by logic; one who is in pain goes to the doctor's office!"

- These same derivations imply that there are limits to these needs. After all, the pious man, whose story stands as the main talmudic source for the obligation to protect one's health, obeyed a higher law and endangered his life in the process.

The Duty to Heal

Providing Medical Treatment as a Religious Duty: Rambam's Approach

Let us now examine the other side of the coin: the doctor's duty to treat, as opposed to the patient's duty to accept treatment. Of the theories seeking the grounding for the duty of physicians to heal, by far the best-known and best-accepted is that of Rambam, who, by no coincidence, was a renowned physician as well as a rabbinic authority. It is first described in his commentary on the Mishna, in the context of interpreting a passage dealing with whether a person who has sworn not to receive benefit from another is nonetheless permitted to medically attend him. Rambam states that such attendance is permissible because it is required:

> And this [person] is not forsworn to [attend in his sickness] the ill person himself because it is a commandment, that is, the biblical obligation of the physician to heal the ill of Israel. This is included in the interpretation they provided of the verse "and you shall return it to him,"[28] to heal his body, that occurs when he sees the other in danger and he can save him, whether in his body, in his wealth, or his wisdom.[29]

The basic obligation to which Rambam refers is the duty to restore lost objects to their owners. The duty is stated twice in the Bible:

> When you encounter the ox or donkey of your enemy wandering, you must take it back to him.[30]

> If you see your brother's ox or sheep gone astray, do not ignore it; you must take it back to your brother. If your brother does not live near you or you do not know where he is, you shall bring it home and it shall remain with you until your brother claims it; then you shall give it back to him. You shall do the same with his donkey; you shall do the same with his garment; and so too shall you do with anything that your brother loses and you find: You must not remain indifferent.[31]

Rambam's innovation does not lie in his applying the concept of "lost property" to the person of the victim; that extension is found in the Talmud.[32] Apparently, the Talmud relies upon a linguistic oddity loaning itself to a *halakhic* pun. The passage in Deuteronomy 22:2 reads, "*v'hashevoto lo.*" This was translated as "you shall give it back to him," but the same words can be taken to mean, literally, "you shall return him to him"—that is, return to your brother his own (threatened) existence. Closely connected to this is the prohibition "do not stand idly by the blood of your neighbor";[33] this verse is cited in the same talmudic passage, establishing a duty of rescue of one who is in danger, and is codified by Rambam as follows:

> Anyone who is capable of rescuing and did not rescue transgresses "do not stand idly by the blood of your neighbor." The same for one who sees his fellow drowning in the sea, or beset by highway robbers, or by a wild beast, who is capable of rescue himself [but does not] . . . transgresses "do not stand idly by the blood of your neighbor."[34]

Understanding that these verses imply a duty of medical care on the part of physicians is novel to Rambam—novel, but not surprising, inasmuch as Rambam's life was so dominated by his medical practice. Novel too, I believe, is Rambam's establishment in the first passage here of what has become known in our times as the "biopsychosocial" model of medical care, a vision of practice that embraces concern for the patient's physical ("in his body"), mental ("in his wisdom"), and social ("in his wealth") well-being.

The Shape and Limits of the Duty to Treat

The very image conjured up by the verses is one that is suffused with a sense of personal responsibility, going far beyond the workaday world. Imagine a physician who treated patients as these verses, in their careful rabbinic understanding, command one to care for lost property: He is never entirely "off call." Should he encounter an emergency outside of working hours, walking along the street, minding his own business, he may not "remain indifferent." His cares are taken along with him at night when he returns home, as the lost object is brought home with him, to care for, as though it were his own object, as though his patient's concern were his own concern.

The nature of this obligation again defines its own limits, for caring for the other as you would for yourself implies not caring for the other any more than for yourself. As a result, fulfilling these laws does not require a total abnegation of the self. An elder walking along need not pick up and care for a lost object in circumstances when he would not pick it up were it his own;[35] you are obliged to care for the object as though it were your own, not more than you care for your own.[36]

These proposed groundings for an obligation to treat share some of the themes that were noted regarding those underlying the obligation to seek treatment. As before, specific biblical injunctions are lacking or at best obscure. The norm is, nonetheless, vigorously upheld, testimony to the feeling that this is a duty taught by logic and common fellow-feeling as well as by Scripture. Throughout, medical care is treated as one among the other contingencies of life, and duties associated with medical care are continuous with other duties of concern for self and for others.

What are the limits to an obligation to heal, grounded in love of the neighbor or the duty to restore lost objects? And, correlatively, is there a limit to an obligation to the self, a point at which the duty to seek treatment no longer obtains? Concretely: What if the lost object has been willfully discarded? What if the patient wishes to die? R Barukh Halevi Epstein is almost alone among rabbinic commentators in drawing what appears to be the logical conclusion:

> "Do not stand idly by the blood of your neighbor": They said of this in TB *Sanhedrin* (73a) "From whence [do we learn] that one who sees his fellow drowning in a river, or mauled by a beast, or beset by highway robbers, is obliged to rescue him? We were taught [by the verse] 'Do not stand idly by the blood of your neighbor.'" That is to say: Do not stand by watching him shed his blood, but rather rescue him.
>
> It is plain that when they say "drowning in the river" this is because it is against his will, just as when he is mauled by a beast or beset by robbers; all the examples are from this same category.
>
> For this reason it should be questioned whether one who intentionally drowns himself, either because of life becoming a burden upon him due to some pain, or because he despairs of life on account of an incurable illness which causes him to suffer,—are we required to rescue him?

And perhaps we may rely upon that which was said in [TB] *K'tubot* [67b] on the topic of charity, that one who has money but is so miserly that he does not wish to be supported from those funds need not be supported from the charity fund, even though he may die of starvation, since that is his own choice; in the same way, here, that is his choice in drowning himself and committing suicide. The matter needs further thought.

In the book B'samim Rosh (attributed to Rosh)[37] section 345 it is written that "one lacking bread and utterly bereft who says before two [witnesses] 'I despair of life,' and who went and committed suicide, did not act as an intentional suicide, nor anyone who acted in this way from his many pains, worries, and suffering or total poverty." (However, I have already written elsewhere [*M'kor Barukh*, introduction, chapter 4] that there is no guarantee that the Rosh in fact authored this work.) And compare *Pitchei T'shuva, Yore Dei'ah,* 345 100b.

That which we described of one who suffers from an incurable, dangerous illness that causes him pain—that we are not obliged to rescue him if we see that he is committing suicide—may be reinforced by the words of Rabbenu Nissim [TB *N'darim* 40a] who wrote, "There are times when you are obliged to ask for mercy that an ill person should die, as when he suffers greatly from his illness and he cannot survive; and so we have seen of the maidservant of R Judah [TB *K'tubot* 104a], who, when she had seen him suffering greatly from his pain, said, 'May it be Thy will that those above should overcome those below,' that is, that he should die swiftly." Now behold: If it is permitted to pray that he should die swiftly, certainly he should not be rescued when he drowns himself in a river on account of his suffering from an incurable illness.[38]

The logic of a regime of duty required R Epstein to pass from a discussion of the limits of the duty to heal (and to rescue) to its correlative, the duty of a person to protect his or her own life. The radical substance of his suggestion—which was, of course, presented very tentatively—will not be pursued further at this time (see Section 4).

The Doctrine of Informed Consent in Jewish Sources

Anyone who has studied contemporary bioethics will be familiar with the centrality of the doctrine of informed consent. At all levels, from introductory undergraduate textbooks to advanced scholarly work in professional journals, discussions and analysis of consent and its associated concepts—standards of information, competence to consent, voluntariness of consent, duration, specificity, and so on—assume a dominant position.

Current Rabbinic Treatment of Informed Consent: Neglect and Repudiation

By contrast, almost no textbook or general compilation dealing with Judaism and bioethics contains a chapter or even an indexed reference to informed consent and its associated concepts.[39] With the single substantive exception of consent to hazardous, nonvalidated medical and surgical treatment (often misleadingly termed "experimentation"; to be dealt with later),[40] the doctrine of informed consent is mentioned only so that it may be dismissed as of any Jewish relevance. The following statements are representative:

> Since one may endanger one's own life no more than anyone else's, Jewish law requires no consent for operations deemed essential by competent medical opinion.[41]

> The first point which must be made is that in Jewish law a person does not have the right to dispose of his body purely in accordance with his wishes: man does not possess absolute title to his life or his body. As a result of this principle, the extent to which the wishes of the patient in question are relevant to the termination of his treatment does not figure in the body of this text.[42]

Medical advice that a given condition is, or may be, dangerous must be heeded. . . . Hence, the patient must seek treatment.[43]

Just as the physician is obligated to heal, the patient is commanded to seek medical attention according to normative standards of behavior. He is not allowed to refuse standard medical treatment.[44]

These brief statements constitute the entire extent of their authors' discussion of informed consent (again, with the sole exception of "experimentation"). Indeed, having said that, there appears to be little more to say about Judaism and consent—except for drawing what appears to be the unpalatable conclusion. Speaking of a patient of the Jehovah's Witness faith who refuses a blood transfusion, Dr. Fred Rosner and Rabbi Moshe Tendler go so far as to write,

If the written refusal to accept blood transfusions is even a psychological debit to the physician or surgeon, then he should refuse to accept the case and refer the patient to another physician. If no other physician is available, or if the Jewish physician accepts such a patient, then the wishes of the patient must become secondary to the command of G-d. If non-Jews are prohibited from taking even an unborn life, surely they are prohibited from taking their own life. For a patient bleeding to death, blood must be administered even in the face of written refusal of the patient. . . . If the physician thereby exposes himself to legal prosecution in violating the instructions of his patient, careful consultation with competent *halakhic* and legal authorities is essential.[45]

The various, overlapping themes reflected in these quotations are set out well in the most complete Jewish treatment of the doctrine that I know; an extended quotation will help set the stage for our further consideration.

Informed consent to medical treatment is a new concept, and as such is not found in *halakhic* works. Also, its valuational bases, by means of which current concepts and parameters of informed consent were expounded, are not by and large appropriate to the view of *halakha,* as will be explained in what follows.

The central principle underlying the concept of informed consent is the value of autonomy. However, the power of this value is limited according to the view of *halakha.* In the *halakhic* understanding, there is a duty upon the physician to heal, and a duty upon the ill person to be healed, and therefore the entire value foundation underlying the principle of informed consent is almost totally nullified. According to *halakha,* the mode of treatment is frequently not established according to the will of the patient and his consent, but rather according to the objective situation. . . . Therefore, regarding an ill person or evident injury, when the doctor has certain knowledge and clear acquaintance, and employs definitive and proven treatment *[refuah b'duka ug'mura],* certainly the ill person who refuses treatment in case of danger is coerced, and [his express refusal] is not accepted; all that is needed to save life is done, even against the ill person's will, and each person is commanded to so act because of [the verse] "do not stand idly by your neighbor's blood," and the matter does not depend upon the view of the ill person. And if there is an ill person in need of an operation to save him, and there is a preponderance [of medical opinion][46] that this operation will succeed, the operation should be done against his will, as long as there is no concern that the mere fact of coercion shall cause him to experience an even greater danger.[47]

The conclusion is clear: There is no role within Jewish tradition for anything resembling the doctrine of informed consent. The premises upon which this conclusion rests are, however, much less clear. They include a peculiarly constrained notion of consent and a distorted vision of the ordinary nature of medical choices. We will examine these problem areas in order, keeping in mind their extremely close interrelations. This leaves us with the challenge of describing what a specifically Jewish doctrine of informed consent, grounded in duty, would look like.

Reading these quotations, one may be left with the impression that the sole value of the doctrine of informed consent is to enable patients to refuse life-saving medical treatment. To be sure, the right to refuse life-saving treatment is commonly understood to follow from the doctrine of consent, but to think the two are identical is an error of almost comical proportions, like identifying your right to vote with the spoiling of a ballot.

Consent in Current Bioethical Theory

In current bioethical discussion, "informed consent" serves as a kind of shorthand for a certain kind of relationship between patient and health care provider.[48] A relationship that respects informed consent is one in which a doctor treats the patient seriously, as a mature, responsible adult with independent values. Acknowledging that the decisions to be reached are decisions about the life of the patient, the doctrine requires that the doctor provide information in the amount and manner that the patient will find most useful in thinking about and, ultimately, deciding upon medical choices.

In this current understanding, the doctrine of informed consent does not speak to a single event—the acceptance or rejection of a specific medical treatment—but rather mandates an extended process of education of, and negotiation with, the patient. As such, the doctrine is not restricted to a single dramatic moment when a patient accepts or declines life-saving interventions; properly understood, it suffuses the medical encounter. When a patient is told that an antibiotic might cause diarrhea, that dental Xrays should be taken, that her backache does not seem serious but she should stay off her feet for a few days, that "this will only pinch a bit"—in all these cases, the values of informed consent are at issue.

The doctrine, therefore, may play several roles, over and above that of protecting a patient's autonomy in critical decisions: It provides an occasion for mutual respect between doctor and patient; it helps to improve medical treatment, by insisting upon two-way communication between doctor and patient; and it promotes, as well as protects, the patient's autonomy, by providing the patient with the tools as well as the opportunity for decision making.[49]

This view of consent recognizes no bright dividing line between medical choices and life choices. It recognizes that the decision of a patient maintained on hemodialysis to undergo a transplant operation is a choice between two ways of life, no less than between two medical procedures. Understanding that the patient within this medical encounter is a person in the full sense, and not simply the spatial locus of a disease process, the doctrine of consent naturally demands that the practitioner adopt a multidimensional, biopsychosocial view of the processes of diagnosis and treatment. And it is a doctrine that remains no less relevant as an inevitable process of dying progresses, even though it appears that the medical options are slim to none, as is evident in the following case excerpt:

ETHICS CONSULTATION: WHY TELL THE TRUTH?

Mr. L, seventy-three years old, had been followed for years for mild bronchitis. He was now admitted to hospital for a minor surgical procedure (transurethral trimming of the prostate). Part of his presurgery workup involved a neurological consultation for weakness in both legs; on the off chance, a CT scan was ordered, and it unexpectedly found several cancerous regions in his brain. Subsequently, a chest film revealed what was probably Mr. L's primary site, in his lung.

Disease is so far advanced that Dr. F does not recommend chemotherapy. However, radiation treatment is indicated, to forestall several likely results of the spread of cancer in the brain: blindness, paralysis, etc. Treatment would be indicated to preserve quality of life, rather than to prolong life per se.

Mr. L has not been informed of his diagnosis or prognosis. His son, a man of early middle years, who is much by the bedside and had accompanied him when seeing the doctor for years previous, insists that his father not be informed. At the same time, he agrees that his father ought to be treated; and for his part, the father appears to have agreed to treatment, under whatever belief or misapprehension he was laboring regarding the intent of treatment. Those treating Mr. L are impressed with his son's intelligence, reasonableness, and warm concern, and so are loath to ignore his wishes. However, the radiotherapists have said that they will not treat unless the patient has himself signed an informed and valid consent to treatment. They also suggested I consult on this.

A meeting of attendings and residents was held prior to meeting Mr. L's son to determine whether he should be told in the event of his continuing resistance to informing his father that the physicians are obliged to provide this information regardless of his wishes.

The son was understood to be saying that the knowledge that he has cancer would kill his father, would make him suicidally depressed. Nobody knew why the son would think this specifically, though one recalled the son's relating that his father had once said, "If I have cancer, that's it, I am dead." It is my belief that the son's feelings, rather than being completely a reaction to his father's ability to absorb the cancer diagnosis, were characteristically Greek, as in earlier consultations, in which impending death was a secret to be kept from family members [see the earlier ethical consultation, "An Offer of Truth"].

The son was also saying that he wants to take his father out of hospital, and take him to his native Greece, for treatment and to spend his final days in familiar surroundings. It was unclear whether this was an idea of his of long standing or a reaction to being pressed to inform the father of his condition. I speculated that the son had thought of this for some time, but had wanted his father stabilized and under treatment before departure, later speeding up his agenda under the spur of the prospect of this information. At the later meeting, the son confirmed this speculation.

There was no question raised by any participant regarding

the basic competence of this patient to understand the nature of his condition and decide about treatment accordingly.

Various views were expressed during the discussion about truth-telling in general and in this situation, including the belief that it is wrong to inflict information about a fatal diagnosis upon someone unwilling to know about this. An important countervailing issue, though, was the fact that, because of the radiotherapists' stance, unless the patient was informed, he would not receive needed treatment. It was not known, however, how much information he would need to be given to satisfy radiotherapy, and the sense was that they might be leaving this up to the clinical ethicist's judgment. There was common agreement that if the patient did ask about what was found, and specifically whether he has cancer, the doctors could not lie to him.

I described briefly my bias in favor of telling the truth, and some of the ethical and legal parameters to truth-telling as that relates to consent to treatment. To be valid, consent must be based upon the information the patient requires to make a choice. The ordinary touchstone is the information the average, reasonable patient requires; but a person may require less information, and can waive information, yet still provide a valid consent. Information and insight should not be inflicted upon the unwilling. When there is a warranted belief that information would be directly detrimental to the patient, it may be withheld under the doctrine of therapeutic privilege, but this is a narrow exception, requiring specific reasons for believing the patient to be vulnerable to disclosure.

A general consensus was reached in favor of a partial disclosure to the father, that a "mass" or "growth" had been found, which could go on to cause symptoms and which should be treated by radiation. The side effects of the treatment would be fully described. This would give him some basic information on which he could make a choice. At least as important, it would provide him an opening for asking further questions, which should then be responded to as fully as he indicates he would want. It was agreed that Drs. F and C and I would speak to the son and describe this proposed course of action.

This further meeting immediately ensued. A long and painful discussion with the son confirmed most of the above information, but added several salient facts. My lack of French forced the meeting to be held in English, in which Mr. L was not entirely fluent. There were difficulties in communication, but my sense was this was caused much more by the nature of the discussion and feelings than by language.

The son described a previous negative experience with a friend who had learned that he has cancer, and eloquently spoke of how dreaded this diagnosis is; he confirmed, as well, that in Greece this isn't spoken of, and his belief that if his father were to travel to Greece and be treated there he would be spared this knowledge. His father is emotionally fragile and has needed to be continually jollied along to accept treatment with a positive attitude.

I was impressed, and made uncomfortable, with three new bits of information the son provided:

· His father has been suffering a good deal of uncertainty about his condition and the information he is being given. He has had, may continue to have, a lurking suspicion that he has cancer and that this information has not been shared with him.
· His father has been asking his son what the doctors have been talking about, telling the son, and keeping from him.
· He is worried that his father would not want treatment if he learns that he has cancer, and this is at least part of the reason he wants this knowledge withheld from the father.

These correspond quite precisely with three main moral reasons for telling the truth and negate the main excuses for withholding the truth about diagnosis and prognosis.

It is commonly impossible to successfully keep the secret from the patient. Patients who are not directly told they are "terminal" usually end up with at least strong suspicions about this. Efforts at secrecy then result in the patient's depression, isolation, and fear, bereft of the opportunity to confront and explore feelings that are natural under the circumstances with the help of open communication with others. The father appears to have entered this state already. This syndrome cannot be dealt with effectively without dealing with its basic cause, the keeping of secrets.

Information about the patient's condition should properly belong to the patient, and be under his control. While a patient may, as noted, waive information, this simply reflects that same right of control. The father has expressed to the son the desire to know what the doctors have learned. Any assertion of this personal right to information must basically be taken at face value. (The son dismisses this desire of his father's as simple curiosity. That is not his judgment to make, or, probably, anyone's.)

Patients require information to make choices reasonably consonant with their own values and desires. As Dr. F had said, disclosing information may not be required in some cases where it will not affect the patient's treatment in any way and where there is a strong countervailing reason. By the son's admission, this is not the case here. Knowing that he has cancer that has metastasized, a patient might reasonably decide to accept radiotherapy or to refuse it; to travel to Greece or to spend what is probably a brief remaining life in Montreal; to leave hospital or to insist that aggressive chemotherapy be attempted. There is a strong temptation to agree with the son that the father might reject treatment and want to go home, and that therefore the information should be withheld. But the moral and legal doctrine of consent is required precisely so that patients will be making decisions, including decisions with which we disagree.

The son has faith in Dr. F's sensitivity and discretion. Dr. F agreed at the close of the meeting to see Mr. L on a daily basis, to be the primary medical spokesperson to the patient, and to coordinate the information he will be receiving. He agreed further to provide Mr. L with the basic information necessary for

Mr. L to make the decisions he faces, but he will avoid directly saying that he "knows" Mr. L has cancer, at least pending the results of a biopsy if that is taken. Dr. F made no commitment to avoid any information that Mr. L needs or wishes to pursue, but will give this information in the most sensitive and gentle way possible.

(My suspicion was that the son and Dr. F were in gentle connivance to pull the wool over the eyes of the ethicist. I had the distinct impression that the son had picked up on the fact that Dr. F—one of the kindest men I've ever known—fully intended to shield the elder Mr. L as much as possible from the truth. If that was the plan, at any rate, it didn't work. The patient insisted, very early in a later meeting with Dr. F, to know everything that was going on. He brushed aside attempts at euphemism, and upon learning that he suffers from widely metastasized cancer, decided to leave the hospital at the first possible moment to return to his native village in Greece. Once there, he said, he will think about whether he wants radiation treatment.)

Implications of the Current View of Consent for Judaism

Questions of truth-telling to the dying patient are seen in this case to be indissolubly tied to informed consent. Consider Mr. L's agreement to undergo radiotherapy: How could this agreement possibly be relied upon, legally or morally, inasmuch as the consent was provided in ignorance of what is being treated and why? For that matter, what possible meaning could this proposed treatment have had for Mr. L himself?

Some may object that I have stretched the concept of informed consent too much, that it should be restricted to communication regarding single, clear-cut, and discrete medical decisions. I would argue with them, for in my view decisions about individual medical treatments cannot be divorced from their context of diagnosis, prognosis, and care—nor, indeed, from the way in which a medical choice fits within, or distorts, a patient's life-plans. But at any rate, if this objection is open to anybody, it is not to one who comes at this question from a perspective informed by Jewish sources.

As we have seen emerging from our examination of the duty to heal and to be healed, whether seen as derivative from a duty to restore lost objects or to never stand idly by when another is placed in danger, Judaism has insisted upon understanding medical care as continuous with other aspects of life, and the obligations that derive therefrom. As we have seen, too, the biopsychosocial model of health care underlying this view of consent was adopted (if not innovated) by Rambam, in his derivation of the duty to heal. The broad view of the doctrine of informed consent is not foreign to Jewish sources; rather, it flows organically from them.

Consider the following analogy. It may be argued on the basis of Jewish sources that a person has self-regarding duties of financial, as well as physical, well-being. A person holds wealth in trust for its true Owner: "to G-d is the earth and the fullness thereof."[50] The wanton destruction of useful objects is prohibited.[51] In addition, persons are forbidden to squander their resources, so that they not become objects of charity, charges upon the public purse. Would it be reasonable to infer from these premises that a person is under a religious obligation to seek out financial counselors and to obey their advice—blindly, unthinkingly, without asking them their reasons? Yet that is the inference drawn regarding medical treatment, on the part of those who deny a role within Jewish bioethics for informed consent. Nor may the analogy be discounted by countering that, religiously, health is of incomparably more importance than financial well-being. Granting, for the sake of argument, that this is so, this might simply imply that one is all the more required to question a doctor's advice, investigate and weigh options, and so forth, than is true of financial decisions.

On the other hand, it may be objected that the authors I quoted earlier (and the many others who could have been cited) never meant to say that informed consent in this broad sense has no role within Judaism. They meant simply to deny an absolute right to accept or to refuse *all* forms of medical treatment. There is some truth to this, although I would state it differently: Writers on Judaism have not recognized the fallacy in reasoning that because consent is not an absolute value, it is therefore of no value at all.

In addition, the silence of these authors is telling. If they understood that there exists a role within Judaism for the doctrine of informed consent in this broader sense, they would have described it, albeit under a different label. The works I have quoted were selected, in part, because of their claims to being comprehensive surveys of the major bioethical issues seen from a Jewish perspective.

The Nature of Medical Choice and Its Implications for Consent

Medical Choice in Current Jewish Sources

A second underlying error on the part of those who see no role for consent within Judaism arises from a basic misunderstanding of the typical medical choice. Because patients are not absolute masters, owners, of their own body—because patients are not permitted to endanger themselves—we are told that there is no role for informed consent. Rather, the authors inform us, a doctor's instructions must be followed; as we shall see later, many go on to add that if the patient resists, then he or she must be coerced: by the rabbinic court if possible, by the doctor if necessary. So much, in their view, for the typical medical choice. Exceptionally, a patient is afflicted with a disease for which no standard treatment has been established, although hazardous, unproven, "experimental" surgery is possible. The case is sometimes posed as one of even odds, "evenly balanced upon the scales";[52] the treatment may cure or it may kill. In these unusual cases, many rabbis acknowledge, the patient may be given the choice of accepting or refusing this unproven treatment, provided other conditions obtain (see Section 4).

It is this rare occurrence that accounts for the discussion of consent, such as it is, in Jewish works; the following statement is typical of this *oeuvre:*

> A patient who is seriously ill and will in all probability die within a short period of time may, on expert advice, and with his consent, be given an experimental drug or other treatment that offers a chance of cure, even if there is also a risk that his life may thereby be further curtailed.[53]

The famous medical adage, taught to every resident, says, "When you hear hoofbeats, think horses, not zebras." In bioethics, as in medicine, the beginning of wisdom lies in developing sound judgment, the ability to distinguish between the usual and the rare. The view of medical choice expressed by many rabbinic authorities that underlies their rejection of a role for consent in Jewish law violates this adage. It posits as ordinary the vanishingly rare; as rare, the usual if not uniform situation.

Here is what the usual medical choice looks like for this view: The patient's illness has been diagnosed correctly and unequivocally by his physician. The diagnosis is objectively, or at least intersubjectively, true, in the sense that all other doctors would arrive at an identical diagnosis. The prognosis is equally certain. There is one single effective treatment for this disease, recognized as such by all other doctors. The treatment is unambiguously indicated; for example, it is without serious side effects. Without the treatment the disease will continue or worsen; with it, the patient will be healed.

This is, at any rate, the current authoritative rabbinic view. Rabbis have not always had such faith in medical judgment. Ramban, for example (echoing Plato), had written that in medical treatment nothing is certain: What cures one patient may kill another (see later).

Consider the following responsum passage, by R Eli'ezer Waldenberg, the most prolific contemporary rabbinic authority on medical law. He writes in response to a question from an Australian rabbi concerning a proposed law mandating psychosurgery in certain cases of childhood mental illness, whether with or without parental consent; central to R Waldenberg's view is the distinction between usual medical choices and the kind of choice psychosurgery might pose:

> In all treatments [generally] even though [it is true that] if the doctor were to err the patient's death will be hastened, nevertheless, the doctor in treating the patient is certain, with the information at hand, that he will by this [treatment] heal the sick person provided no complication occurs, and only if he makes a mistake the treatment will kill the patient; unlike a

treatment as at present, regarding which even current medical information testifies that it is itself potentially lethal ["a potion of death": *sam hamavet*] and may kill the sick person; and the doctor from the very beginning, armed with current medical knowledge, begins with this doubt: If he does not cure him, he may kill him.[54]

It is clear why, given this view, there is no role assigned to patient choice in the typical case. If a medical recommendation is objectively right, definitively in the patient's best interests, who needs patient choice? At best, a patient will accept the recommendation; in that case, consent is redundant. Alternatively, the patient will refuse the recommendation, in which case the patient has sinned.

The Realities of Medical Choice and Uncertainty

But this view describes the rescue fantasy of patients far better than the felt reality of practicing physicians. From the doctor's point of view, every aspect of care is riddled with uncertainty, guesswork, creative insights that leap beyond the evidence, and conscious as well as unconscious trade-offs. Diagnosis is almost always presumptive, rather than conclusive, and at each point in medical investigation there always remains more that could be done to refine the diagnosis: a new test to run, an old test to check. Every treatment option carries with it the risk of side effects, which need to be weighed against the risks associated with alternative treatments and the risk of not treating at all. Treatment recommendations are constantly shifting, in response to factors ranging from new clinical studies to reimbursement patterns and patient demand. Many current standard treatments have never had their safety and efficacy scientifically established; some, which have been validated, are soon superseded by new and promising treatments or cast into the shadow of previously unsuspected late-onset side effects.[55]

These uncertainties lead to tremendous differences that have often been noticed in the way in which medical practitioners in different regions treat similar kinds of patients. As David Blumenthal writes,

Fifty years of scholarship have established the existence and importance of the variation phenomenon in modern medicine—the observation of differences in the way apparently similar patients are treated from one health care setting to another. . . . [It is not realistically] conceivable that all patients with the same condition would be treated in precisely the same way in every place, by every provider, and at every moment. The variation phenomenon is an indicator of a fundamental fact of life that many physicians recognize: the daily practice of medicine is a huge, ongoing natural experiment, the results of which await our measurement and interpretation so that the knowledge gained can be put to constructive use.[56]

These points should be familiar and obvious. Consider the two most common causes of death by illness today, heart disease and cancer.

The detection and treatment of early heart disease are suffused with controversy. Some hard diagnostic information, like a patient's cholesterol level, is easily obtained, but its significance is uncertain and at best can contribute to a probability judgment. Whether this information should be cause for medical concern, and in what fashion—diet, drugs, exercise—is equally shrouded in controversy. Those firm recommendations that do emerge—lose weight, don't smoke, and so on—are grounded much less in knowledge than in a prudent guess: not because "this will definitely help" but rather because "this can't hurt." The management of late heart disease, like myocardial infarction (heart attack), is surrounded with the same doubts, although there, of course, the stakes are much higher. Who should be hospitalized, and for how long? What medications should be given, in what doses, and when? Who should be treated surgically, who with medication?[57]

Many of these same uncertainties are reproduced in cancer. The detection and management of precancerous conditions, or conditions predisposing to cancer, are major sources of dispute. The relative effectiveness of the alternative forms of treatment for established cancer is unresolved, whether taken singly or in combination. Whether we speak of surgery, radiation treatment, or chemotherapy, the same set of questions recur: how? where? how much? when? for whom? In addition, and contrary to R Waldenberg's claim that only rarely does a doctor commence treatment knowing it might kill, all cancer treatment is fraught with risk. Indeed, our current chemotherapy is effective in precise proportion to its danger.

Yet another factor confounding a physician's ability to predict is that of patient variability in the course of disease and in reaction to treatment. The rabbinic rejection of a role for patient choice rests upon a two-sided conditional: If the patient is treated, he will be healed; if not, he will languish, worsen, or die. The medical uncertainties noted here, combined with patient variability, ensure that this conditional judgment can never be made with confidence. The point was graphically, and tragically, demonstrated in a widely publicized case in Israel. An elderly woman in Tiberias, suffering from advanced gangrene of the leg, had refused the recommended amputation; as she put it, she chose to enter Paradise on her own two legs. A personal visit and appeal to her by the Sephardic Chief Rabbi of Israel convinced her to agree to the amputation. She underwent the amputation, and died within days of surgical complications. The case is almost a tailor-made demonstration of the fallibility of medical judgment.

R Moshe Feinstein, a rabbinic authority distinguished for the depth of his compassion as well as his learning, acknowledges the factor of patient variability in the following excerpt; yet even he fails to recognize how it, coupled with other sources of medical uncertainty, eliminates as a practical matter the rabbinic basis for coercing patients to undergo medical treatment:

> Question: Are we required—or, to what extent are we required—to compel a sick person to receive against his will medicine or treatments or even investigations in order to identify the illness. And what if there is in the medicine itself some danger (of course, less than the danger of the illness).
>
> Answer: The case in which the ill person does not wish to accept treatment depends upon whether this [refusal] is because he despairs or whether it is because he is in pain and

considers that just at this time he does not wish to be in pain—even though he believes the doctors [who claim] that this is for his benefit, that he will be healed thereby, or that they will know from this how to heal him. This is a childish, irrational act—they must compel him if this is possible for them. However, if it [his refusal] is because he does not believe these doctors, then they must find him a doctor in whom he does believe; and if there is no such doctor and it is impossible considering his illness to wait until he understands that this is in his benefit, nor to send him (should he desire this) to doctors and a hospital in another city, the physicians here are required to act against his will if all the doctors in this hospital are of the view that this is his treatment. In addition, this must be accomplished in a manner that will not frighten him, for if he will be afraid of this, even for an illogical reason *['inyan shtut]*, then it is not to be done; for fear can harm him and even kill him, and it would be as though they had killed him with their own hands. Therefore, it is better not to do this against his will, even though that is what the relatives desire.

The physicians need very much to study the matter whether to compel him when it occurs that an adult ill person does not want treatment and it is probable that it will not be very helpful, and to do this only for the sake of Heaven [i.e., only when they are scrupulously certain that their intention is proper]. Moreover, if the medicine itself poses some risk but the doctors are accustomed to give this medicine when the patient has a dangerous illness, even though the danger of the medicine is much less than that of the illness, then under no circumstances should the patient be compelled.

In addition, intrinsically, regarding giving a risky medicine like this, which physicians are accustomed to give when the ill person's illness is more dangerous than the medicine: The knowledge that physicians have from those who are healthy or mildly ill, or simply weak, in whom we find that they are not as deeply endangered from this medicine that they wish to give to this ill person on behalf of his serious illness—we should conclude nothing from such events; and therefore such a risky medicine should not be given, for it is possible that for this ill person it poses a great danger. Only when the doctors know that even those who have this sickness, and are weakened to this degree, have also not been endangered by the medicine except for a very small minority— then, when the doctors are of the view that no less than half of ill persons have been healed, are they permitted to give this medicine when he has the status of an ill person; and the doctors must have much consultation on this among many and great physicians present there, for this form of estimation is very difficult, even for great physicians.[58]

The Proliferation of Medical Choices

One final factor warrants discussion. We noted earlier the mistake in identifying the doctrine of informed consent with the right to refuse life-saving treatment. The same mistake recurs on the part of those rabbis who presume that medical knowledge has advanced to the point of posing a binary choice: Accept treatment and be healed; refuse treatment and deteriorate. For it is rarely the case that there is only a single form of treatment available. The form, manner, and timing of treatment are far more often matters for negotiation, and rarely can be conclusively settled by a scientifically justified medical recommendation. Even when the major questions of diagnosis and modality are settled, after all, some, albeit circumscribed, choices remain open: between, for example, this antibiotic, which often causes diarrhea, and that one, associated with allergic reactions.

All too often, the field of choice is tragically open, and it defies reason to think that one and only one therapeutic approach is "medically indicated." One well-explored example of this is the management of patients in end-stage renal failure. Should the patient be treated on dialysis or seek a kidney transplant? The advantages of transplant, provided of course a suitably matched donor organ is available, are formidable: better quality of life, fewer dietary restrictions, and others; above all, no longer needing to be tied to a kidney machine for hours on end, twice a week. But the choice may not be

clear for all, particularly for one whose body has already rejected a do-
nated organ.[59] There are surgical risks, and risks of antirejection drugs,
associated with transplantation. A patient on dialysis is also spared the
emotional roller coaster ride in store for a patient on a transplant list.
On reflection, even an "objective" choice between dialysis and transplant could not be attempted without taking into account the patient's own life patterns, plans, and values. The routine of dialysis is
psychologically tolerable for some, but impossibly claustrophobic to
others—and for some, as a purely practical matter, the routine is occupational suicide. The doctrine of informed consent allows these
medically relevant factors to come out in conversation between doctor
and patient, so that an appropriate therapeutic plan may be imple-
mented.

I presented the treatment choice for patients in kidney failure, for
clarity's sake, in an artificially simplified form. In reality, many more
options present themselves: hemodialysis or peritoneal dialysis? with
or without erythropoietin? cadaveric transplantation or a donation
from a near relative?

The following case illustrates how, in another context, the field of
choice ramifies.

Ethics Consultation: Cancer in Pregnancy

Mrs. M is a twenty-one-year-old married woman who is
twenty-five weeks pregnant with her first child. She presented
with unexplained anemia that grew progressively worse, without
explanation despite investigations. This week a definite diagnosis of recurrence of cancer in bone marrow was made. She is
now pancytopenic, and very likely would have died already had
she not received treatment and blood products.

A short time previously, she had a form of cancer, medulloblastoma, that is usually found in children. She was surgically
and oncologically treated and was told—as her surgeon believed—that she was cancer free. She was worried that she had
not waited long enough after radiation before becoming pregnant, and that the baby might be damaged. The baby's condi-

tion seems fine, though, and it is of normal size for gestation.

My initial phone contact with Dr. Q, Mrs. M's obstetrician, indicated no conflict between the interests of the mother and baby, probably because of the absence of treatment options for the patient; but at that time he hadn't yet spoken with an oncologist. That there is no conflict no longer appears to be the case, but many uncertainties remain. There is no good data on treatment and survival for a recurrence of this unusual cancer in adult patients. One survey article on recurrence that the patient's family doctor (Dr. N) had reviewed gave two-year survival rates of 0% untreated, 46% treated; but nobody believes the figures would be anything like that optimistic for this patient. Treatment would presumably be aggressive chemotherapy, including vincristine.

The patient's social status compounds the tragedy. A Muslim married to a Hindu, she had been disowned by her own family and is not approved of by her in-laws (with whom she and her husband live due to financial constraints). She very much desires this baby, and both Drs. P and M were of the opinion that her priority is the baby rather than her own life. She is aware that she is very ill. That day she had been informed that ultrasound revealed the baby is probably female, and expressed worry that after her death her in-laws might put up the baby for adoption since, in her words, "a girl is a curse on a Hindu household."

There has not been any conflict between Mrs. M and her husband with respect to giving the baby priority, but that might change; he had that day or the previous day asked about how soon treatment could begin—it wasn't clear to me whether he said this knowing treatment would probably require delivery of a premature baby whose chances are compromised. The patient herself is well-oriented, intelligent, aware in a general way of her condition. She delays dealing with some information because of what her doctors judge to be an appropriate defense mechanism to the sudden alteration in her prognosis.

A lengthy discussion ensued. The primary questions dealt

with were aimed at arriving at a treatment plan and deciding how choices might be expressed to her and made by her. (Also discussed were legal and ethical questions associated with late abortion/early delivery, ethnic and religious factors, etc.) The discussion proceeded on the assumption that Mrs. M does indeed want to save the baby, even at some risk to herself, possibly grave risk; but some direct means of verification that such are indeed her wishes may be needed, under contingencies as indicated here.

It was agreed that we would try to track and respect her desires; at the same time, it was agreed that the stark choices of a mother's vs. a daughter's life are impossibly difficult and need to be presented to her as treatment recommendations rather than as a cafeteria of options with associated probabilities of risk to her and her baby. Because our efforts will be to track her own views rather than to impose medical views upon her, we considered and rejected a proposal to present the risks (to mother and fetus) of all the alternative treatment options to the oncologist and have him express a treatment recommendation on that basis.

The next step at this time is to ascertain whether there exists a genuine conflict between mother and infant in recommencement of treatment. Pending that, it was also agreed that for the interim, should Mrs. M's condition deteriorate drastically and suddenly, the baby would immediately be surgically delivered by caesarian section.

The oncologist should be asked these questions, in this order:

- If Mrs. M were not pregnant, should cancer treatment begin? (It is possible that the chances of success are so small that treatment would not be indicated.)
- Under the same assumption, is it prudent to delay treatment for several weeks?
- And if not, is it prudent to begin therapy with agents not

toxic to the fetus for a period of several weeks, and later switch to more aggressive therapy?

In the event that toxic cancer treatment would be immediately advised were there no pregnancy, it becomes imperative to verify the belief that Mrs. M is prepared to undergo some substantial risk on behalf of the safety of the fetus, and then to proceed on that basis.

Further discussions may then be needed. The obstetrician described the likelihood of intact survival of the fetus if delivered now as lying in the neighborhood of 50%. If the fetus were instead to be delivered by caesarian section in three weeks' time, the chances go up a great deal, perhaps approaching 90%. A further delay, to thirty-two weeks, enhances the chances further—95%?—but the feeling expressed by those participating in this meeting was that such an extended delay is hitting the law of diminishing returns. It did not receive much further consideration. Also considered was whether it was possible that the baby's chances might in fact be enhanced by early delivery, vs. continued gestation in a compromised host; at present there is no such indication.

Finally, the issue of resuscitative measures and code status for Mrs. M was also discussed with Dr. N as something that will need to be addressed with Mrs. M, perhaps after the current issue is resolved.

[Postscript: Discussion between Mrs. M and her doctors confirmed that she wished above all else that her baby be saved, at whatever risk to herself. The oncologist consulted on this case with physicians from the world's leading center of expertise on this cancer, who felt that early and aggressive chemotherapy would not substantially contribute to Mrs. M's survival. Shortly thereafter, Mrs. M "crashed," and an emergency delivery was done. The mother did not survive this medical crisis. The baby appeared to be healthy and undamaged and went home with its father, with the full support of his extended family.

Contrary to all expectation, however, a tumor was found on autopsy to have infiltrated the placenta, and the baby will have to be monitored closely for signs of medulloblastoma.]

Why Has Rabbinic Literature Failed to Acknowledge Medical Choice?

In brief: The absence of a rabbinic doctrine of informed consent is predicated upon the view that, in general, the patient's illness is diagnosed with certainty, and medical knowledge dictates that illness be treated in a single manner. This view, which fails to take seriously both medical uncertainty and medical controversy,[60] is so obviously false, so contrary to what every medical student is taught, that one wonders how it became so engrained in rabbinic thought. A number of possibilities suggest themselves. Rabbinics, no less than medicine, is a full-time job, and those rabbis writing on medical ethics rarely have any medical training or professional exposure to health care settings. Rabbinics is a profoundly conservative enterprise, and contemporary writers often rely upon beliefs that were widely held hundreds of years past. Here is a paradox, for only with the scientific grounding of medical practice, largely a phenomenon of the latter half of the twentieth century, has it become common to publicly admit the facts of medical uncertainty and controversy. In earlier times, when the most powerful thing a physician had going was the patient's belief in the physician's knowledge and efficacy—the basis of the placebo effect[61]—it might be (quite literally) lethal for the patient to learn of the physician's misgivings.[62] It was then, at a time when medical authority was most firmly (and groundlessly) insisted upon, that rabbinic beliefs regarding medical certainty solidified.

In addition, it is plausible to speculate that rabbinic confidence in medical knowledge was bolstered as the result of a positive feedback loop. Disclosing uncertainty and controversy is, for many treating physicians, awkward and inconvenient: a chore that might be required by law or professional norms, but not a rewarding part of medical practice. These physicians, treating a (rabbi) patient who has been acculturated to believe implicitly in his doctor's wisdom, are unlikely to disabuse the patient of his fond illusions. And the more this happens, the more likely are rabbis to believe in their physicians, and the more likely are physicians to feed this belief; and round and round.

It is, at any rate, an illusion. Diagnosis is uncertain, prognosis indeterminate, treatment options shrouded in controversy. (One further factor, the multiplicity of treatment goals, will be addressed in Section 4, on risk.) It is almost never the case that a doctor may justifiably tell the patient: "Here is the situation: Do what I say, and live; resist it, and die." Whether and how to respond to a test result or a presenting complaint represents an exercise in weighing risks and benefits: a prudential judgment, if not out-and-out guesswork. To this judgment, the patient's input is essential: his history, pattern of life, plans, and values. And the modern doctrine of informed consent is the framework permitting that input to be provided.

An Alternative Construction: The Reasonable Caretaker

The Duty of Self-Care Applied to Persons

Let us return to first principles in developing an alternative paradigm for understanding a role that informed consent might play within the Jewish approach based upon duty. The verses discussed earlier that were understood to establish a duty for a patient to seek medical care state that persons must "take care *[hishameir],*"[63] must indeed "take great care" *[v'nishmartem m'od],*[64] of their souls (i.e., their lives). The Hebrew verb root common to these verses is *SHMR,* a term whose semantic range includes the ideas of caring for, guarding, keeping safe. The person charged with this act, with safeguarding, is called a *shomeir:* in English legal jargon, a bailee. I shall refer to this *shomeir* as a "caretaker." In the rabbinic understanding of these verses, then, they call upon persons to act toward their lives as toward an object they are solemnly charged to safeguard.

Prominent among the explanations for Judaism's neglect of (indeed, rejection of) the concept of informed consent is the view that a person has no "ownership" *[ein ba'alim]* over his own body, his own life. If "owner" there be, that owner is G-d. This is another way of establishing the same point: Persons are in the position of *shomrim*, caretakers, vis-à-vis their physical well-being. From this point of view, what appears as a duty to (one's own, physical) self may be seen as a duty to the Owner of that self. Duties to that Owner are of necessity *mitzvot*. As R Moshe Chayim Luzzatto writes,

> This too is a *mitzva* upon us, to safeguard *[lishmor]* our bodies in a fashion appropriate to enabling us to serve through it our Creator; and we should make use of the world with this intention and towards that end, as we may require.[65]

The Duty of Self-Care Extended to Patients: A Case Study

What follows from this relationship? It has been taken for granted that if persons do not own their bodies, they have no rights over them; and hence, they can have no right to informed consent.[66] But for that very same reason, persons have duties with respect to the body, duties to act as prudent caretakers. Because of the nature of the "relationship" between a person and his or her body, nobody else can understand precisely what medical treatment will mean better than that same person. Hence, *only the patient can truly fulfill the demands of bodily preservation and caretaking.* And that duty cannot be properly fulfilled without the exercise of informed choice regarding medical treatment.

ETHICS CONSULTATION: AMPUTATION

I was contacted by phone by Mrs. C on Monday, April 2, regarding her father; she had apparently gotten my name and the idea to call me from a mutual friend. Her call concerned her father, Mr. N, ninety-four years old, who had been admitted the previous Wednesday for fever. Apart from other medical conditions (Parkinson's, hernias, etc.), Mr. N has bad peripheral circulation, and had begun to develop a gangrenous spot on his toe seven months earlier. He had been assessed by a vascular surgeon (Dr. T), who had recommended an arterial graft. The graft had not been performed at that time. The call concerned medical choices for Mr. N; I agreed to meet her the next day.

Tuesday from 1—2:30 or later I met with Mrs. C, her brother, and the patient, her father, Mr. N, in the emergency room. I spoke as well with Dr. D, the physician on service in the emergency room, and briefly with the senior attending physicians available, Dr. G (internal medicine) and Dr. L (geriatrics).

In spite of the lengthy discussions, the questions were really quite clear. These family members had experienced difficulty in reaching a decision because of their inability to receive medical information about the choices from the surgeon, Dr. T. They wanted to know the answers to such questions as: How long would recuperation take? Could it wait until after a family celebration (the wedding of Mr. N's granddaughter) in June? Could it wait until after he could no longer walk upon the foot? Was he well enough to survive the procedure? Why was an above-the-knee amputation recommended rather than something less? I was only of limited help, e.g., in clarifying that although the condition had been described to them verbally as "dry gangrene," in fact Dr. T had written on the chart his clinical sense that it is "wet" (that is to say, infected, and relatively more urgent). The chart indicated that Dr. T's clinical judgment was probably confirmed by laboratory results. I discussed with them what would likely follow if the gangrene was infected.

In addition to this need for information, though, the family needed clarification about who was the decision maker here. Both daughter and son accepted in principle that their father was competent to decide regarding this amputation—that this was not the son's, but rather the father's, decision to make; but the son had difficulty in putting this understanding into practice.

The patient was an observant Jew who was lying quietly on his cot in the emergency room reciting from the Book of Psalms. At the time that I spoke to him, he was drowsy and did not seem to understand everything that was being said. However, he was generally responsive and stated that he needed time to think about this. I left having expressed concern to Mr. N and to his family members that if the patient does not decide fairly soon to go ahead with the procedure that he may be discharged. Other than surgery, there is no treatment he is receiving in the hospital that he could not receive back home.

The case of Mr. N, absolutely routine in so many ways, reinforces some of the points argued here regarding the nature of medical choice. Despite tests and follow-up, there remained uncertainty about the diagnosis and, consequently, the prognosis. Not a single choice, but numerous options, were on the table: not just "amputate or not," but also "amputate—when?"; "amputate—how much?"

Behind the scenes, there was medical controversy as well. The elusive Dr. T has a specialty in vascular surgery. Despite his excellent technical reputation, many of his colleagues consider him too quick with the knife, particularly regarding geriatric patients. Dr. G, the internist, has worked with Dr. T over many years, and says that "he is right more often than not"; Dr. L, the geriatrician, feels that a ninety-four-year-old patient with a number of intercurrent diseases should think more than twice before agreeing to this. Dr. D, the emergency room doctor, distances herself; she just wishes everyone would make up their minds already, so she could either arrange Mr. N's admission to the surgical service or discharge him.

In the rabbinic view, there is no role for consent because the patient must accept the doctor's recommendation. But there is no "doctor" here; rather, there are too many doctors. Nor is there a medical recommendation; rather, there are too many such.

Even more than these lessons of uncertainty, however, this case demonstrates how the medical choices must be resolved by the patient, for only he can understand their implications within the context of his own life. Mr. N is an elderly, sick, pious man. He uses his legs to get up and walk to synagogue services daily. He would like to attend his granddaughter's wedding; he would like, for that matter, to attend the circumcisions of his great-grandchildren, if he could be spared that long; but he would also like to enjoy and be as active as he can in whatever time he has left. What should he do, as a reasonable caretaker of his physical self? How best will his current medical choice express his duty to safeguard his life?

Can a doctor tell him what he should do? Hardly. Dr. T, the surgeon, who is himself the most convinced of all that he knows what is the right treatment for Mr. N, will not, as a matter of principle, operate unless Mr. N himself wholeheartedly agrees to the operation. As a surgeon of the old school, Dr. T takes it as a matter of faith that patients who are forced under the knife do poorly. As a humane doctor, Dr. T is also quite aware that there is little point in operating if Mr. N is not prepared to fight through an arduous period of rehabilitation. Mr. N's will to live, his determination to fight, are facts that only Mr. N himself is privileged to know, as is the depth of his pain. Dr. T would agree with the rabbinic interpretation of the verse in Proverbs that states that only the patient's "heart knows its soul's bitterness."[67] Dr. T recognizes that only through speaking with Mr. N—telling him of what can be done, and what this will mean for Mr. N's life—can a rational treatment approach be discovered. If this is true for Dr. T, how much more so for the other treating physicians? for the family members? for any rabbi who happens to be asked what the Law requires of Mr. N?

Mr. N told me that he needs time to think about this. He is absolutely right. He is a caretaker of his body, holding it in trust to fulfill his obligations to his fellows and to his Maker. If he were entrusted with a large sum of money on behalf of another, he would have to carefully study before deciding what he should do with it: stuff it in his mattress? put it in the bank? invest it? As a reasonable caretaker of another's property, he would have to consult with experts in financial management. He would have to consider their advice carefully, ask questions, perhaps seek second opinions; but in the end, he would have to decide, because it is him to whom the money was entrusted. He may do no less regarding his own physical person.

Legal Implications of the Duty to Care for the Self

Jewish law recognizes several different classes of *shomrim*, caretakers. A person may be a *shomeir* of an object he has borrowed from another, for example; he may, on the other hand, be paid to look after an object; he may need to care for an object he has rented. These forms of caretaking have diverse laws of liability; for example, one type of caretaker is liable to repay the owner in case of theft, another is not. But there is one form of liability common to all caretakers: *p'shia*, negligence.

A caretaker who has failed to meet this common denominator of liability has committed *p'shia* with regard to the entrusted item. It is, therefore, at least suggestive to note the same language being used regarding one who has failed to properly safeguard his own life and health; he is said to be *poshei'a b'nafsho*, "negligent concerning his soul" (i.e., as noted earlier, life), or *poshei'a b'gufo*, "negligent concerning his body." Among those guilty of this form of negligence are those who refuse to seek medical attention—"Anyone who is careless in this and relies upon a miracle is akin to being self-negligent"[68]—as well as one who became ill as a result of failing to take necessary precautions.[69]

What is the legal standard of *p'shia*? What measures must a caretaker take to avoid being negligent with respect to the entrusted object? The principle established in the Mishna[70] is that "every caretaking not done in accordance with the custom of caretakers *[k'derekh hashomrim]* is negligence." In the absence of any special agreement or undertaking to the contrary,[71] the abstract basis of negligence and responsibility requires that persons who assume a social role undertake to perform it with at least the degree of care routinely assumed by any other average person similarly situated in that society. The same reasoning and associated standard underlie the law of professional liability in common law. For example, a physician must act as would an average, reasonable practitioner.

This abstract principle must, of course, be fleshed out by means of example:

If he wrote to the other, "send it to me with whomever you choose," and he sent it to him and it was lost, or the agent denied the claim, he is inculpable *[patur]*, provided he sent it by a trustworthy person and in the manner by which persons are accustomed to transport their assets. However, if he sent it to him by means of one who was proven to be untrustworthy [*kafran*], or through a dangerous route, that most are not accustomed to use for the transfer of assets, he is negligent and culpable.[72]

The standard of negligence established by the rabbis is, in the first instance, relative to the nature of the object being guarded. Proper precautions for a load of bricks will not suffice for a shipment of gold, and the care suitable for gold bullion will not be appropriate for fine china.[73] The standard is also one that is avowedly relative to time and place. Indeed, the Talmud's discussion of the Mishnaic principle of *p'shia*[74] itself indicates the point; at one time, the Talmud writes, money could be stored under the roof beams or between the bricks, "but now that there are housebreakers, now that there are rappers" who look for loot by breaking the beams or rapping on the walls for hollow sounds, the law requires new hiding places. This "progress" did not end with the sealing of the Talmud; as conditions and customs change, actions that were negligent in eighth-century Babylonia, for example, may be perfectly acceptable now, in North America.[75]

One fascinating eighteenth-century responsum, rich with historical detail, discusses a woman who had moved to Jerusalem. The people of her home city had entrusted her with items for delivery to relatives in Jerusalem. The rabbi author describes approvingly the precautions she took while aboard ship, and how, upon arriving at Sidon harbor and being informed that Jerusalem is full of thieves (!), she realized that her precautions were not sufficient for this changed circumstance. With the assistance of her maid, she opened her locked chest, and sewed the most valuable objects to her undergarments.[76]

Mr. N is caretaker on behalf of his own body. What steps does he need to take to ensure its proper care? As in other cases of caretaking, all is relative to the time, and place, and custom of those similarly situated. As applied to the amount of information he is obliged to request and assimilate in choosing whether, when, and how to undergo an amputation, Jewish law requires him to seek out and utilize that amount of information that would be demanded by the average, reasonable patient, at that time and at that place, facing a similar diagnosis, prognosis, and options.

Consent in Jewish and in Secular Law: Duty or Right?

As it happens, this is the same standard that has been adopted by many common-law courts in the United States and Canada. The old rule had established a "reasonable practitioner" standard. Reasoning that the task of informing a patient is a professional act, like prescribing medication, a doctor needed to tell a patient that information which the average, reasonable doctor would provide to a patient similarly situated. But this reasoning had ignored the fact that the point of providing information is to enable a patient to decide what to do on the basis of that information. Therefore, in many jurisdictions this has been superseded by the "reasonable patient" standard: A doctor needs to supply that amount of information which the average, reasonable patient finds necessary in deciding whether to undergo the treatment in question. A doctor who has fallen short of that standard is in breach of the duty to gain the patient's informed consent.[77]

On one level, the similarity between this new common-law approach and the standard that may be derived from Jewish sources is strong. Much effort has gone into clarifying precisely what a "reasonable patient" standard means, in terms of disclosing risks, benefits, and other sequelae of a procedure and its alternatives. Case law has been accumulating for more than twenty years, dealing with the application of the standard on a very practical level. For example: Is a doctor obliged to provide advice, his or her best judgment, as well as information?[78] Is a doctor obliged to describe statistical information about life expectancy associated with a recommended treatment?[79] At the same time, a voluminous bioethical literature has burgeoned, providing a more theoretical treatment of the problem.[80] These rich discussions can help inform our understanding of what Jewish law requires of a patient.

On a deeper level, we should recognize that the underpinnings of the common-law approach and those of Jewish law are radically divergent. In common law, a patient has a right to information; correlative with that right, a physician has a duty to supply it. In Jewish law, a patient has a duty to be informed, as a necessary preliminary to the obligatory exercise of proper trusteeship over his or her own body. In a common-law approach, a patient may waive the right to be informed—that right is the patient's, to do with as he or she may choose.[81] When, as in Jewish law, informed consent is the patient's duty rather than right, the patient is morally obliged to fully engage in the interaction that is informed consent: consulting with health care providers, asking questions, exploring alternatives, and so on.

If we look at this another way, we will see that the gulf between the common law and Jewish approaches is even deeper. As a right, informed consent is but one side of the coin, with informed refusal on the other side. It is impossible, as a matter of the logic of moral concepts, to speak of one who has a right to accept treatment but no right to refuse treatment. That is undoubtedly one important factor underlying the rabbinic rejection of informed consent. A right to consent to needed medical treatment entails a right to refuse it. Such a right is inconsistent with the obligation to preserve the integrity of the body held in trust for its Maker.

The reasoning process is, however, erroneous, for the same logical correlativity of consent and refusal does not hold for consent considered as a duty of patients. The patient-physician interaction in fulfillment of a patient's duty of informed consent will be quite similar to that undertaken in a common-law jurisdiction in respecting a patient's right; yet no element in this duty entails that the patient has the right to refuse beneficial treatment. To see this, a final basic difference between the moral logic of a regime of rights and one of duties needs to be clarified.

For our current purposes, the duty of informed consent can be broken down into two major components. First, the patient must seek out that information relevant to the task of caring for the body and must attempt to understand the information gathered, in relationship to the patient's own life and life-patterns. Second, the patient must employ that information in practice by reaching a reasonable decision regarding treatment options. The first task is the "informed" component of "informed consent"; the second, the "consent" component.

Both components are subject to the patient's option in the regime of rights. A patient may or may not choose to become informed, and may or may not agree to any form of treatment. *But neither component is optional in the Jewish regime of duties.* A patient is obliged to become informed and is obliged to consent to that form of treatment (or non-treatment) that the patient finds is best suited to the obligation of caring for the body.

Consent as a Duty and Coerced Consent: The Resolution of a Legal Paradox

The "consent" component therefore plays different roles in the two regimes. In the regime of rights, consent is an *unconditional, free option*. In that of duties, consent is a *power*. This power is not unconditional: It must be exercised in accordance with Jewish law. Nor need this power be freely exercised: Within the Jewish legal regime, consent that has been coerced may yet be effective. Yet the act of consent itself retains its necessary legal force.

Some explanation is required of this legal provision that departs quite radically from the common law (and indeed, from Roman law itself).[82] In Jewish law, the fact that a person had consented under duress does not invalidate the consent. To take the graphic example provided by the Talmud, if a merchant were hung by his neck by a customer until he agreed to sell[83] some item, the sale is nonetheless valid.[84] Jewish law, unlike more familiar legal systems, sharply differentiates between the commercial transaction, which is validly effected by the consent provided, and broader considerations of social policy, punishment, and criminal law.[85] While the sale is valid, the customer will be subjected to the full rigor of criminal sanctions for his actions. Yet the consent itself (in the form of an agreement to sell) is no charade, or mere legal form. If the property were forcibly stolen, and subsequently an agreement to sell were extracted by duress from the merchant, the transfer of property is legally void.[86]

How do these points apply to consent to medical treatment? I am not, of course, suggesting that a doctor is permitted to coerce patients to undergo treatment. The license to coerce is one that is held by a court alone, and even then, only under stringent conditions. The point is introduced because of its theoretical importance. If we think of patients as caretakers of their persons rather than as free and unfettered individuals, we may then understand informed medical choice as a power of a patient, rather than as a patient's right. In this construct, the idea of a coerced consent is not a contradiction in terms, and the theoretical possibility of a court's coercing a patient to accept treatment does not mean that the patient's consent was "never really" needed.

To illustrate, let me furnish two further examples of the phenomenon of coerced consent; the first is found in Jewish law, the second in Jewish theology. The legal example is drawn from the realm of divorce. By biblical rule, only the husband is entitled to divorce his wife. The rabbis, however, recognized many grounds upon which a wife may present a valid claim to a divorce: for example, mental or physical abuse. What is to be done when a woman has a valid claim to divorce, yet her husband refuses to sign a bill of divorcement? The rabbinic rule is, "He is coerced until he says, 'This is what I want'" [kofin oto 'ad sheyomar rotze ani].[87] The husband's consent to divorce is, in the Jewish regime, by biblical decree, a real power; his agreement is a necessary condition for a divorce, but this power is not unconditional—he is morally obliged, by Torah law, to grant his wife a divorce under specified circumstances—nor need it be freely exercised.[88]

The theological example underlies the entire structure of Judaism, the covenant at Mount Sinai between G-d and the Jewish people:

"And they stood beneath the mountain":[89] R Avdimi son of Hama son of Hasa said, This teaches that the Holy One Blessed be He placed the mountain above them like the cover of a bowl and said to them, If you accept the Torah it is well, and if not, here shall be your gravesites.[90]

"I aroused you beneath the apple tree":[91] Palti'in of Rome expounded, saying: Mt Sinai was plucked up and placed standing in the high heavens, and Israel was placed beneath, as it says "And you came near and stood beneath the mountain."[92]

The idea that consent may be coerced is, of course, incomprehensible in a regime of rights. Not so in a regime of duties. In this second case, for example, consent is itself necessary to the establishment of a covenant, but since the Jewish people were duty-bound to accept that covenant, it was morally acceptable to compel that consent and to act upon it once compelled.

Consent in a regime of duty, then, plays a real role, but one very different from that which it plays in a regime of rights. Nonetheless, because of medical uncertainty and other points noted here, it remains the case that even within a Jewish regime the duty to consent leaves the patient with the need to weigh a variety of options of treatment (and nontreatment). In the next sections, we shall examine Jewish sources that describe who may be entrusted with the duty to safeguard the person (Section 3, "Competency") and in what manner that duty is responsibly performed (Section 4, "Risk").

Endnotes

1. *Sefer Hachinukh,* attributed to R Aharon Halevi.

2. See C. J. McFadden, *The Dignity of Life: Moral Values in a Changing Society* (Huntington, IN: Our Sunday Visitor, 1976).

3. Compare with 2 Kings 4.32 and 2 Kings 5.8.*

4. Ex. 15.26.

5. II Chron. 16.12.

6. Abraham Ibn Ezra, Commentary on Ex. 21.19.

7. Ramban, Commentary on the Torah, on Lev. 26.11.*

8. See Onkelos's Aramaic translation of the verse *v'agar asya y'shaleim;* Onkelos on Ex. 21.19.

9. TB *Bava Kamma* 85a.

10. *Akedat Yitzchak, Vayishlach,* Gate 26.

11. Lev. 18.5.

12. TB *Yoma* 85b; TB *Sanhedrin* 74a.

13. J. David Bleich, *Contemporary Halakhic Problems 2* (New York: Ktav, 1983): 55, claims this view was held by R Shimon ben Tzemach Duran (*Teshuvot Tashbetz* 3, section 37).

14. Deut. 4.9.

15. Deut. 4.15.

16. TB *Brakhot* 32b.

17. See R Barukh Halevi Epstein's Torah commentary, *Tora T'mima,* on Deut. 4.9, note 16.*

18. Maharsha, TB *Brakhot* 32b.

19. On Deut. 4.9 see R Moshe Chayim Luzatto, *The Way of G-d*, beginning of chapter 1; p. 30 in Arye Kaplan, translation, 4th revised edition (Jerusalem: Feldheim Publishers, 1983).*

20. Alhough not unknown; see *Shir Hashirim Rabba*, Chapter 8, v 3.*

21. See *Minchat Chinukh*, Commandment 546, section 11.*

22. *Mishne Tora, Hilkhot R'tzicha Ushmirat Hanefesh*, 11.4.*

23. TB *Sh'vu'ot* 36a.

24. Rambam, *Hilkhot Sanhedrin*, 6.3.

25. Gen. 9.5.

26. TB *Bava Kamma* 46b.

27. Fred Rosner, "The Physician and the Patient in Jewish Law," in *Jewish Bioethics,* eds. Fred Rosner and J. D. Bleich (New York: Hebrew Publishing Company, 3rd printing, 1985): 54.*

28. Deut. 22.2.

29. Rambam, *Peirush Hamishnayot, N'darim* 4.4, s.v. *hamudar hana'a meichaveiro.*

30. Ex. 23:4.

31. Deut. 22: 1–3.

32. TB *Sanhedrin* 73a.

33. Lev. 19:16.

34. Rambam, *Hilkhot R'tzicha Ush'mirat Hanefesh* 1.14.

35. *Shulchan Arukh, Choshen Mishpat* 263.

36. Some have claimed that Ramban (Nahmanides) used another source for the duty to heal, namely, the commandment to "love your neighbor as yourself" (Lev. 19.18). They base this on his discussion in *Torat Ha'adam* (in *Kitvei HaRamban* II, ed. Bernard Chavel, [Mossad Haravkook Jerusalem, 5724]: 43). I discuss this in Section 4.*

37. R Yitzchak ben Asher.

38. R Barukh Halevi Epstein, *Tosefet Brakha* on Lev. 19:16.*

39. See, for example, compiled and edited by Abraham Steinberg, MD, from the works of R Eli'ezer Waldenberg, *Jewish Medical Law* (Woodmere, NY: Beit Shamai Publications, 1989); Prof. Abraham S. Abraham, *The Comprehensive Guide to Medical Halakha* (Jerusalem: Feldheim, 1990); Fred Rosner, MD, and Moshe Tendler, *Practical Medical Halakha*, 3rd rev. edition (Hoboken, NJ: Ktav, 1990); J. David Bleich, *Judaism and Healing* (Hobo-

ken, NJ: Ktav, 1981); Fred Rosner, *Modern Medicine and Jewish Ethics* (Hoboken NJ: Ktav, 1986).

40. Compare with Immanuel Jakobovits, *Jewish Medical Ethics* (New York: Bloch, 1975): 291 ff.

41. Immanuel Jakobovits, "Judaism," in *Encyclopedia of Bioethics,* ed. Warren T. Reich (New York: Free Press, 1978): 799.

42. Daniel B. Sinclair, *Tradition and the Biological Revolution* (Edinburgh: University of Edinburgh Press, 1989): 4.

43. J. David Bleich, *Judaism and Healing* (Hoboken, NJ: Ktav, 1981): 23.

44. Compiled and edited by Abraham Steinberg, MD, from the works of R Eli'ezer Waldenberg, *Jewish Medical Law* (Woodmere, NY: Beit Shamai Publications, 1989): 23; following R Eli'ezer Waldenberg, Responsa *Tzitz Eli'ezer* 4, section 13, paragraph 2; *Ramat Rachel* sections 20, 21; 11, sections 41, 42.

45. Fred Rosner, MD, and Moshe Tendler, *Practical Medical Halakha,* 3rd rev. edition (Hoboken, NJ: Ktav, 1990): 164.

46. Compare with Responsa *Tzitz Eli'ezer* 4 section 13, end.*

47. "Informed Consent *(haskama mida'at),*" in *Entziklopedi'a Hilkhatit-R'fu'it,* vol. 2, ed. Dr. Avraham Steinberg (Jerusalem: Falk-Shlesinger, 1991): 1–47, at 22–25.

48. See Robert J. Levine and Karen Lebacqz, "Informed Consent in Human Research: Ethical and Legal Aspects," in *Encyclopedia of Bioethics,* ed. Warren T. Reich (New York: Free Press, 1978): 754–762; Jay Katz, *The Silent World of Doctor and Patient* (New York: Free Press, 1984); Howard Brody, *The Healer's Power* (New Haven, CT: Yale University Press, 1992).*

49. This framework was introduced in Jay Katz, Alex Capron, and Eleanor Glass, *Experimentation with Human Beings* (New York: Russell Sage Foundation, 1972).

50. Ps. 24.1.

51. Known in Jewish law as the principles of *bal tashchit.*

52. See, e.g., *Tzitz Eli'ezer* 4, section 13.

53. Abraham S. Abraham, MD, *The Comprehensive Guide to Medical Halakha* (Jerusalem: Feldheim, 1990): 147.*

54. Responsa *Tzitz Eli'ezer* 4, section 13.

55. The reasons why medical diagnosis is suffused with uncertainty should be elaborated upon at greater length than I can provide here.*

56. David Blumenthal, "The Variation Phenomenon in 1994," *New England Journal of Medicine* 331 (1994): 1017–1018.*

57. Blumenthal (1994).*

58. R Moshe Feinstein in *Halakha Ur'fu'a* 4, ed. R Moshe Hershler (Jerusalem: Regensburg Institute, 1985): 111–112. See also Daniel Sinclair, "The Status of Medicine and Medical Treatment Against the Patient's Will" (in Hebrew), *Sh'naton Hamishpat Ha'ivri* 18–19 (1982–1984): 265–294.*

59. See Lee Foster, "Man and Machine: Life Without Kidneys," *Hastings Center Report* 6, no. 3 (1976): 5-8.*

60. The rabbinic view ignores as well the possibility of medical error, a factor that deserves at least a passing mention.*

61. See Howard Brody, *Placebos and the Philosophy of Medicine* (Chicago: University of Chicago Press, 1980).

62. Consider, e.g., many passages in Molière's play *Le bourgeois gentilhomme.**

63. Deut. 4.9.

64. Deut. 4.15.

65. R Moshe Chayim Luzzatto, *The Way of G-d*, 1.4.7.

66. Compare with Steinberg (1991).

67. Proverbs 14.10; TB *Yoma* 83a; Rambam, *Sh'vitat ha'asor* 2.8.

68. R Eli'ezer Waldenberg, Responsa *Tzitz Eli'ezer* 8, section 15: *Kuntres M'shivat Nefesh*, ch. 16, s.v. *harachaman hu;* similarly, in his volume 10, section 25, s.v. *perek shloshim.*

69. Responsa *Yechave Da'at* 4, section 14, s.v. *ume'ata navo.* For another example of usage, see *Tur Orach Chayim* 37.*

70. TB *Bava Metzi'a* 42a.

71. See *Tur Choshen Mishpat* 290, 291: A *shomeir* can choose to assume more stringent responsibilities than *p'shia.*

72. *Tur, Choshen Mishpat* 121.*

73. See *Tur, Choshen Mishpat* 291. Compare further on this standard *Tur, Choshen Mishpat* 176 and 290.*

74. TB *Bava Metzi'a* 42a.

75. See, e.g., Responsa *Minchat Yitzchak* 6, section 166.*

76. Responsa *Admat Kodesh* 1 *Choshen Mishpat* 73.

77. Among the early and influential cases to establish a reasonable patient standard is *Cobbs v. Grant,* 502 P. 2d 1 (Cal. 1972).

78. *Zamparo v. Brisson,* Ontario Court of Appeal, 1981, 32 OR (2d) 75–85.

79. *Arato v. Avedon,* 858 P. 2d 598 (Cal. 1993).

80. Among the more significant treatments are included Jay Katz, *The Silent World of Doctor and Patient;* Tom L. Beauchamp and Ruth Faden, *A History and Theory of Informed Consent* (New York: Oxford University Press, 1986); Paul S. Appelbaum, Charles W. Lidz, and Alan Meisel, *Informed Consent: Legal Theory and Clinical Practice* (New York: Oxford University Press, 1987).

81. *Reibl v. Hughes,* Supreme Court of Canada, 114 DLR 3d 1-35, Oct. 7, 1980, per Laskin CJ; Benjamin Freedman, "The Validity of Ignorant Consent to Medical Research," *IRB: A Review of Human Subjects Research* 4, no. 2 (1982): 1–5.

82. See R Isaac Herzog, *The Main Institutions of Jewish Law,* vol. 2 (The Law of Obligations, 2nd ed.) (London: Soncino Press, 1967): 130–131.*

83. For a sale to be valid in Jewish law it must satisfy both substantive and procedural requirements.*

84. TB *Bava Batra,* Chapter *Chezkat Habatim,* 47b ff.

85. The broader philosophical implications of this stance must await clarification on another occasion.*

86. See Rambam, *Mishne Tora, Hilkhot M'khirah,* Chapter 10, law 5.

87. TB *Arachin* 21b.

88. In the case of sales as well, Jewish law has established that compulsion does not render an agreement ineffective; cf. TB *K'tubot* 109b.

89. Ex. 19.17.

90. TB *Shabbat* 88a; compare TB *Avoda Zara* 2b; compare TB *Bava Batra* 40a.*

91. Song of Songs 8.3.

92. Deut. 4; *Shir Hashirim Rabba,* on 8.3.

COMPETENCY

jewish sources and the general theory of competency

Introduction

Among the most contentious issues in a society that values freedom is that of establishing freedom's boundaries. The political and legal system's first recourse is to the rule of law: The scope of free action is constrained by the establishment of laws and regulations. Some actions are designated as criminal: They are stigmatized, and their perpetrators are punished. Others are controlled by the civil law system: They are regulated, and their perpetrators are subject to financial sanctions.

Another approach is needed, on behalf of that segment of society whose behavior seems immune to the first form of control. Included here are children and the mentally ill or intellectually handicapped. On the one hand, being unable to conform their conduct to law, it seems both futile to expect them to be law-abiding and unfair to punish or to fine them for their failures in this regard. On the other hand, their actions, unfettered by criminal and civil laws, can result in damage to themselves and those around them. The second form of social and legal recourse is therefore to limit the freedom and effective autonomous action available to these persons designated as incompetent for these purposes. This form of control may be effected in a number of ways, including the appointment of guardians to act on behalf of the incompetent person and the close physical supervision and even control of the lives of incompetents.

Competency's Role in Allocating Social Power

In this chapter, I will particularly focus on a third form of social control, the nullification or adjustment of the legal consequences of the choices and acts of incompetents, in particular, the mentally ill. By definition, this form of control is socially relative, varying according to the kinds of roles, responsibilities, and rights that a given society expects of its members. All societies face a variety of decisions about competency, that is, about which persons will be allowed to freely assume and exercise a social role: competencies to contract, to bequeath property, to marry or to divorce, to judge or to be judged, as well as to consent to medical treatment. And each delineation of competency must be responsive to the social context within which the role will be fulfilled: Competency to contract means one thing in a barter economy, something very different in one that trades in stocks and bonds. Yet underlying these differences there exists a common core of questions that any society faces in deciding to restrict the effective action of some of its members. Some of these questions are contained within the following case.

ETHICS CONSULTATION: DRUNK AND BIPOLAR

Mr. U is a sixty-seven-year-old man with a lengthy history of bipolar disorder (previously called "manic-depression"). He has been an alcoholic since his twenties. He has held responsible business and management positions despite these conditions, which have necessitated repeated hospital admissions over the years. His psychiatric condition has been controlled on lithium. His last admission, when he was brought in by police in a very confused state, resulted in the discovery that his kidney and liver functions are failing, under the dual onslaughts of his medication and drinking.

His daughter has been the sole person from the family caring for him and has effected his hospital admissions in the past. She is exasperated at having this responsibility without the power to effect change between these clean-ups. She wants to be appointed curator over his finances, and she wants him to be treated as an inpatient.

Dr. P did the psychiatric assessment of competency. At that point in time, Mr. U, who had been taken off lithium for a period to allow his organ function to stabilize, was nevertheless as clear cognitively and as stable in reaction as he had ever been. Mr. U told the psychiatrist he will try to drink less after release, but admits that this good intention is likely to remain unfulfilled. As a sixty-seven-year-old man, he feels that there is not that much time left to him, and he may as well spend it enjoying himself in taverns in his accustomed pattern. Remarking on Dr. P's skiing injury, he asked, "Did you ever think maybe you shouldn't ski? Should someone stop you from skiing and hurting yourself?"

I met with Mr. U for about forty minutes. He was easy to spot: He was sitting on the edge of his bed, with a baseball cap on his head, looking for all the world like a geriatric schoolboy waiting for the bell to ring. We talked about some of the events that preceded his hospital admission—his drinking, his profligacy, the time the police were called because he was tossing his collections of phonograph records and of sculptures (*stone* sculptures!) off of his balcony. He said that these just seemed to be the right things to do at that time—time to clean up his house, as it were—and anyway he had never been out of control: He looked down from the balcony to make certain nobody would be hit when he started flinging out the sculpture collection. He understood that his daughter was acting out of her love and concern for him, but at the same time cautioned me—quite plausibly, I thought—not to be conned by the selfless role she has assumed, when she is looking after her own personal and financial interest as well. He was adamant that these choices, for better or worse, are his own to make; and his choice now is to leave the hospital.

His statements regarding his medical condition seemed to me less appropriate. He is not worried about resuming drinking, because he denies feeling anything wrong with his kidneys or liver. When told that the tests he had taken can indicate organ damage before a patient experiences any symptoms, he said that he did not believe the tests could have showed anything wrong.

I discussed with Dr. P the question of Mr. U's competency, and what might follow from that regarding decisions about his treatment. Whereas Mr. U is at this time cognitively unimpaired, he is not, in the longer view, functional. Dr. P had written, but not yet sent, a letter to the Curator of Persons [the government office charged with the authority to order treatment for persons it rules incompetent to decide for themselves]. The letter detailed the fact of the bipolar condition and alcoholism. It noted that when examined the patient was competent, but further stated that the future, given his repeated hospitalizations and occasional profligacy with money (he had spent $12,000 in September, largely on presents to a barmaid), was predictable. With that kind of story, Dr. P's experience suggests, the office of the curator will probably grant the daughter her requested curatorship. Such a decision would be in derogation of the current (quite narrow) legal notion of competency—indeed, it would contradict Dr. P's specific statement that Mr. U was competent when assessed! But the Curator of Persons often takes more factors into account in this assessment than are specifically stated in law. Such action is the curator's choice, and Dr. P, we agreed, is not responsible for doing more than sending in an accurate report.

Another psychiatrist with whom Dr. P had spoken didn't see what all of this agonizing was about. Given Mr. U's history of repeated psychiatric hospitalization, this psychiatrist stated, he was obviously incompetent. Dr. P responded that in the case of another patient, with no diagnosis of bipolar disorder but who experiences severe alcoholism, the same history of treatment could have resulted; yet in such a case everyone would agree that the patient should be discharged as soon as possible, even if the patient wanted to stay—let alone, as here, when the patient wants to leave.

Assuming he is incompetent, though, what decision would be in his best interests? It is still possible that the frustration and discomfort that he would experience as a patient treated by involuntary psychiatric hospitalization would result in Mr. U's lengthened quantity of life at a disproportionate loss of quality of life. Were that the case, perhaps his decision should be respected in spite of his incompetence. There is another, preferable, practical alternative. He is at present euthymic [neither manic nor depressed] and will have an appropriate maintenance dose of medication reestablished shortly. When discharged from the hospital, he will not need closely supervised

treatment. Nor does his daughter necessarily want him confined to a psychiatric facility against his will for a prolonged period of time. What is indicated, rather, is some form of
supervision that would allow for a timely intervention when he
is bingeing or off medication and in an undoubted state of incompetence. Dr. P will ask the social workers if there is some
group home or other setting that would serve this function, in a
way satisfactory to both Mr. U and his daughter. This would
represent, under the circumstances, the least restrictive alternative that would adequately respond to Mr. U's occasionally
urgent needs.

Current Approaches to Competency
in Secular Law and in Medical Practice

A variety of approaches to defining competency to consent to
treatment may be extracted from court decisions, a number of which
have found their proponents within the bioethical literature. Perhaps
the most widely accepted definition has it that a patient is competent
to consent to a given treatment provided he or she is able to understand and appreciate the nature and consequences of the proposed
treatment and its alternatives. In an important review of approaches
to competence, Roth and his colleagues describe, at one extreme, an
alternative definition of competency that requires that the person not
simply understand the choice but in fact reach a reasonable decision;
at the other, one that judges competency provided only that the person express a choice without regard to what the patient understands
that choice to mean or what reasoning process the patient used.[1]

More recently, several versions of a variable concept of competency have been proposed;[2] in this conception, competency requires
progressively greater intellectual capacity as the stakes of a choice rise.
In the variable conception proposed by Drane, for example,[3] patients
are competent to accept those treatments objectively in their best interests provided only that they do in fact consent on the basis of a bare
general "awareness" of their medical situation and choice. At the other
extreme, competence to refuse a treatment objectively necessary to
preserve life, in Drane's view, requires that a patient must not simply

demonstrate understanding and appreciation of the consequences, but, in addition, must provide a rational choice that flows from an intelligible value system.

The diversity of views on competency results from a struggle between opposed, even polar, concepts and values regarding the social role of the mentally ill. The most obvious of these is a conflict between freedom and protection. In the last case, for example, Mr. U was experiencing the double-edged sword that is mental illness. On the one hand, he has not been blamed for his actions. His erratic behavior, so harmful to himself and his family (especially his daughter, the only family member who has taken responsibility for him), has been excused on account of his psychiatric condition. On the other hand, he has had his liberty restricted and faces lengthy if not permanent loss of control over his own financial assets.

Underlying that opposition, in part, are opposed concepts of mental illness. Is there a radical disjuncture between the mentally ill and the rest of us that justifies two basically different social goals—for the ill, protection; for others, freedom? Or is mental illness, a phenomenon at least as variegated as mental health, to be marked along the continuum of human behavior? Mr. U's finger, pointing at Dr. P's leg cast, was pointing (in another sense) to such a conceptual continuum.

Another aspect is the opposition between the perceptions of mental illness and the evaluation of competency as between the settings of the clinic or hospital, on the one hand, and the courtroom on the other. Within a courtroom, the question of competency is adjudicated at a particular moment in time, in binary fashion: yes or no, competent or not. The way in which a court or legal tribunal directly evaluates the competence of the person in question—through testimony, which is to say, talking—slants the focus of investigation toward communication and cognitive capacity. Judged in a health care setting, by contrast, competence may appear to fluctuate over time. It is more/less—or getting-better/getting-worse—rather than yes/no. It is evidenced by the behavior of the person in question, as expressed in a variety of situations. The underlying values of the two institutions differ as well.

Within our society, the court is the bulwark of freedom; the hospital, of well-being. Thus, the biases of the two institutions regarding the polar choice protection/freedom are opposed. The court is most concerned that freedom not be unjustly restricted; the clinical setting, that needed assistance not be withheld.

Competency's Recurrent Social Challenges

While our understanding of mental illness is constantly evolving, the value questions raised by these polar choices are not new at all. As it happens, they are implicit in the numerous Jewish discussions arising regarding the *shote* (pronounced "show-teh"), a person incompetent by reason of mental illness (in rabbinic Hebrew, *shtut*), as well as those incompetent for other reasons (for example, the *peti,* a person with a severe intellectual handicap; children; and others). A rigorous construal of these rabbinic sources demonstrates an approach to competency that is in some ways parallel to current approaches; in others, substantially more sophisticated than contemporary discussion.

I shall describe three components to the theory of competency: first, the minimal conditions of competency; second, competency as an aspect of social policy as well as the logic of human action; third, questions of competency and control as raised in cases of mental illness. I shall cast a broad net, including a variety of forms of competency outside of the medical context. This is a necessary choice in light of the Jewish source materials available. As we saw in the previous chapter, the very concept of consent to medical treatment itself has scarcely been acknowledged by Jewish authorities. This forced choice may at the same time be a welcome corrective to current bioethical literature, which has a tendency to treat medical choice in unrealistic isolation from other life choices.

A caution: As has been often noted before, I intend this book to do no more than provide a foundation for one Jewish approach to bioethics. Accordingly, I will not focus here upon puzzling cases in competency and how to resolve them in practice. Rather, the following remarks are intended to explore the concepts underlying competency, without which those puzzle cases will never be truly clarified.

Competence and Communication of Choice: The Minima

First Precondition for Consent: Consent as a Public Performance

Consent to medical treatment is a public event, in two senses. First, the object of consent cannot be an action performed alone, in private. Consent to treatment implies two persons in coordinated action. Persons do things, but it would do violence to the meaning of the term to say they "consent" to those actions they themselves perform. We can only consent to actions done by others; therefore, the treatment that is the object of consent cannot be "private" action.

Second, consent requires public expression, at least in the form of communication between those same two parties. A patient who has mentally agreed to a physician's proposed treatment has not consented until the physician has been told of this agreement. Nor is this simply a matter of requiring evidence that consent has taken place. Imagine a person who mentally ponders the choice of treatment/nontreatment, going back and forth several times before finally opening his mouth and telling the physician to go ahead. This consent may have been ambivalently given (although it need not be, if the patient reached at the last a firm decision). Throughout this silent struggle, it would be correct to say the patient had withheld consent. But the mentalist account of consent would instead require us to describe this, oddly, as a case in which the patient had withdrawn consent numerous times before reaching a final decision.

These points seem to me logically entailed by the concept of consent, but I will not insist upon that point: It is enough if we agree that this is what we mean by consent in practice. It follows that for a person to be competent to consent, as one minimal condition, he or she must be capable of meaningful communication.[4] Some of the most tragic bioethical dilemmas concern the care of patients who are mentally intact but in a locked-in state, utterly paralyzed, and hence unable to communicate their wishes.

ETHICS CONSULTATION: PONTINE STROKE

Following an earlier discussion with the nurse specialist and the attending physician, a meeting was held with a number of members of staff, myself, and a cousin and two of the closest friends of the patient, Ms. M, to discuss treatment goals and, especially, the decision to continue nutrition [artificial feeding] and hydration [intravenous fluids]. This patient, who had suffered an earlier cerebral vascular accident [stroke], had experienced a pontine stroke while on vacation abroad in the summer and was transported to our hospital, where she was found to be in a locked-in state. Neurology consultation has confirmed the diagnosis and its accompanying irremediable prognosis.

At the earlier discussion, the patient's medical situation had been reviewed, as were statements of her significant others to the effect that she had repeatedly stated her opposition to being kept alive if she should have a disabling disease. These persons wished all life-prolonging treatment, including artificial feeding, to be discontinued. At that time, however, final confirmation that no efforts to establish communication could be successful was not present. The stroke need not have damaged Ms. M's cognitive functions. A consult with Ms. T, from speech therapy, who has experience with communicating with patients with profound physical disability, was to be arranged. All agreed that ideally the patient should decide her course of medical treatment; this required, however, long-term, reliable communication.

Following that consultation, the meeting was held. Ms. M's medical situation was unchanged. The speech therapist has found despite her efforts that reliable communication cannot be established. The patient currently has no acute illnesses, and is not receiving anything other than maintenance care. She had not prepared a mandate [the legal form within Quebec for a person to arrange for medical decisions to be reached during incompetency]; while active, alert, and determined, she had never concerned herself much with legal affairs. Her friends and cousin recounted a number of instances in which Ms. M had stated that she did not wish to be maintained alive in the event of incapacity. While the situations described were not fully comparable to her current situation, these informants felt that they were relevant, in that Ms. M's primary motivation was to avoid being kept alive in circumstances in which she is dependent upon others. (In fact, it was clear to them that Ms. M did not wish to survive in circumstances far better than her current one, or in the situation she would be in after any and all conceivable rehabilitation.) Her friends and cousin were united in this view, having given it lengthy and serious consideration, and related that other friends, unable to attend this meeting, were of one mind on this as well.

While perhaps cognitively intact, Ms. M was necessarily incompetent by reason of her inability to communicate. In the absence of a mandatary or spouse, decision making for an incompetent adult by our law resides in "near relations or persons with a special interest"; those present fulfilled the intention underlying this clause well. (Ms. M's closer relative, a sister, lives in France. She is herself disabled and unable to be involved.) These proxies are charged by law with reaching decisions in the best interests of the patient and consistent with her previously expressed wishes. Reasonable persons can disagree regarding whether continued nutritional and hydration support, necessary to prolongation of life, might be required by, consistent with, or contrary to, the best interests of a person in a locked-in state. There was no question that the patient's previously expressed wishes were contrary to prolonging her life in this state.

The original attending physician, morally opposed to decisions to abate life-sustaining treatment, had asked Dr. D to attend the meeting and assume care of Ms. M. He discussed briefly the approach that he would take: In caring for her he would provide treatment necessary for comfort rather than that designed to prolong her life—including feeding and fluids. It was agreed that, in addition to the health care team, her friends and cousin should tell Ms. M of the meeting and the decision reached. In the unlikely event that there is any indication that the patient rejects this resolution, a repeat evaluation and meeting would need to be held.

Patients experiencing profound paralysis are said to be "locked in" because they are, in effect, trapped in their own bodies. There are any number of possible causes for this condition: As here, there could be a stroke in the pons region of the brain (a common pathway for all voluntary control over movement) or trauma causing similar damage, or it could appear as the last step in one of several diseases destroying voluntary control of muscles (motor neuron diseases, e.g., ALS, or amyotrophic lateral sclerosis). The pressure felt by family, friends, and the health care team when discussing treatment options for these patients is absolutely unique. The patients, for all we know, are fully aware of everything happening to them. Their thinking and sensory capacity—including the ability to feel pain—is also, for all we know, unimpaired. Although we have no way of speaking to a patient like Ms. M, we act in the knowledge that were we to reach the wrong decision we would not simply thwart the patient's previous desires (as may have been expressed in a living will) or have erred in construing what she would have wanted. We would in fact be frustrating her actual, present—but unexpressed and inexpressible—desires.

Second Precondition for Consent: Consent as the Expression of Choice

The ability to communicate is one minimal component of competence. Here is another: Because consent involves the choice of medical treatment, for persons to be competent they must, as a second minimal condition, have reached a settled choice that they will then communicate. An impairment in the ability to decide is a second way in which a person may be unable to play the social role that is consent to medical treatment.

ETHICS CONSULTATION: CRITICAL INTERVENTIONS
IN A PATIENT WITH ADVANCED MULTIPLE SCLEROSIS

The patient, Ms. V, is a woman in her forties. She has had a
lengthy and stable course of multiple sclerosis until a recent ex-
acerbation. Living independently at home, she was admitted to
hospital in the early summer and has gotten worse in spite of repeated courses of treatment on steroids. Last week, when I was
initially contacted, her condition, and particularly the weaken-
ing of her intercostal [chest] muscles, was so bad that a decision
regarding ventilation was considered imminent. It was for the
purpose of clarifying Ms. V's status with respect to critical interventions, especially resuscitation, that this consultation was
held. After meeting with the head nurse and with Ms. V's neurologist, Dr. N, I spoke with Dr. H, who has been Ms. V's psychiatrist for many years and who had seen her the previous day.

A family meeting had previously been held, which by all accounts had gone badly. Ms. V has two parents and a sister who
have been visiting frequently. She has, in addition, an ex-
husband, who joined the picture just prior to my being called,
and two grown children, with whom she has not had contact for
years.

The main decision makers for Ms. V until this point have
been her parents. This burden lies heavily upon them, and it
has become clear that there is some nuance of split, with the
mother more prepared to let go and the father relatively more
insistent upon continuing treatment, including introducing
ventilation, as long as he can still speak with his daughter.
There had not been a sustained effort to ascertain Ms. V's own
wishes. Dr. H's opinion was that Ms. V was cognitively capable
and verbally adept, but whether she would actually be able to
render a decision—something with which she had problems a
long time since, and which had been a theme of her psychotherapy over many years—he thought improbable. Her medical condition compounds this difficulty. While she can speak, her
weakened chest muscles make this a great effort for her.

I spoke with Ms. V in the presence of her neurologist, trying to present her with the simplest possible choice. I told her
that there were medical decisions that might need to be made,
that until this point the staff had mostly been dealing with her
parents, that she was entitled to be the decision maker if she
chose, and that the nature of the decisions were very personal,
so that if she can deal with these matters herself that might be
best. The question: Should we deal with her or with her parents
in explaining the medical options and getting a decision; or,
alternatively, does she want this to be left up to the physician to
do as he deems best?

She began crying as I spoke, and seemed to withdraw somewhat. I asked her if she wanted to think about this and speak to
me later, and she said she did. At the close of speaking with her,
I told her she can take as much time as she wants, but there is
one problem that needs to be answered now: The doctors would
like to do a blood test now to see if an infection has been interfering with the steroid treatments. She readily agreed to this.
Her ability to deal with this simple matter, coupled with her inability to deal with the more serious question of ventilation,
spoke to me of a significant emotional component governing
her reactions.

I met after that with the patient's nurses, and then with her
parents, telling them what was going on, saying that I would return later that afternoon, and that Ms. V should have a chance
to rest before I returned.

I returned that afternoon. Ms. V had not had a chance to
rest, and she was unable to do anything more than that morn-
ing. For the following day, I asked to be kept informed and to
be called when she is ready to talk. A nurse should specifically
ask her, when nobody else is around to influence her, whether
she recalls me and wants to speak with me again. Unfortunately,
her mother was present when she was asked this the next day,
and Ms. V said she was not ready to speak with me again; the
mother was seen shaking her head to the question before Ms. V
said this.

I met the following day with the neurologist, Ms. V's parents, and her sister. The neurologist was concerned about his patient's agitation, and had written in the chart that Ms. V is not capable of dealing with medical decisions now and should not be approached further on these matters. This was his decision to make, although I said that if she asked to speak with me herself, I would of course be obliged to see her. The previous day, when I was not present, an hour had been spent with the patient to explain and receive her consent to a PEG procedure [allowing for tube-feeding]; this was finally done with the assistance of her sister, but Ms. V's own attention span and memory, not to mention emotional state, were too bad to deal with any less clear-cut medical decisions.

Third Precondition for Consent:
Consent and Common Language

A third, minimal condition of competence became evident in this case as well. The physician who is proposing treatment, and describing alternative treatments, needs to have some assurance that the patient is, in at least a general way, aware of what is being asked. This follows, perhaps, from the realization that consent entails communication, for communication implies two persons who have gone beyond mutual gesture or vocalization—who have, in fact, achieved a common language. Despite her intelligence, Ms. V's condition, physical as well as psychiatric, called the existence of this "common language" into question. Also, at the time all this was going on, her energy level was so depleted, and her memory so poor, that by the time a procedure could be described to her in the very broadest of terms, she was too tired to speak, and by the time she had regained her strength, she failed to remember the previous discussion.

A Jewish Paradigm for Competency's Prerequisites:
Competency to Divorce

These three minimal conditions (or prerequisites) for competence—common language, choice, communication—are implicit in a talmudic discussion of a husband's competence to divorce his wife by instructing others to write on his behalf a bill of divorcement—a *get*—and give it to her. It is in the context of divorce law that many discussions of competency in Judaism arise. The underlying Jewish theory of competency, therefore, has to be in large part extrapolated from the case of a husband's competency to give a *get* or a wife's competency to receive a *get*.

Why divorce? Within Jewish society, the single most common form of legally binding contract to which an adult would be a party was a contract of marriage, the *ketuba*. This *ketuba* is an instrument of finance as well as of family law. Developed within a patriarchal society whose overwhelming expectation was that persons would live as part of a marital unit whose husband possesses preponderant financial control, the contract of entry into marriage was required by the rabbis to describe the provisions for financial recompense to which the wife is entitled in the event of divorce. The most likely case in which a court would be called upon to rule regarding the enforcement of a contract would, therefore, concern divorce, at which time the financial clauses of the original *ketuba* would be activated.

The following talmudic passage should therefore be fundamentally understood as constituting an inquiry into legal competency:

Mishna: One who became speechless *[nishtatek]*, and they said to him, Let us write a *get* for your wife, and he inclined his head: They examine him three times. If he says of no, "no," and of yes, "yes," then they write it and give it.[5]
Gemara: Let us be concerned that perhaps he suffers a tremble of "no, no"; or if not, a tremble of "yes, yes." [Rashi explains: A form of madness, that accustoms him to always shake or nod his head, and he is not responding to the words they ask him.]
    —R Yosef bar Manyomei said, We speak to him in stages. Yet we should be concerned that perhaps he has a tremor in stages!
        —We ask him one question of No, and two of Yes, and two of No, and one of Yes.
They learned in R Yishmael's school: They speak to him of

summer matters during winter [the rainy season], and of winter matters during summer.

——What does this mean? Were we to say, of warm winter garments or cool summer garments, we would be concerned lest he is seized by a chill or a fever.

————Rather: of the fruits.[6]

The barrier to competency here is one of communication: The party instructing the preparation of a contract, the husband, has "become speechless" in some manner left unspecified—wisely so, since the salient issue is the absence of communication, rather than the cause of the absence. (Although the term used, *nishtatek*, consistently refers to imposed speechlessness in rabbinic Hebrew—its root, *SHTK,* means "silent"—it has in modern Hebrew acquired the meaning of "paralysis.")

There is no reason to suspect the husband of any form of incompetence or derangement other than his speechlessness, just as was true of Ms. M, the victim of a pontine stroke, although in both cases, it is possible that uncommunicativeness does indeed mask a loss of mental capacity. The case presented follows, and stands in contrast to, a discussion of a case of a man who, seized by *kordiakos* (by the Talmud's description, an acute confusional episode, perhaps caused by alcohol), asks for a *get* to be prepared. In that case, of incompetence due to a patent loss of mental capacity, the Mishna rules the husband's action a nullity.

Unpacking the Prerequisites to Competency: Communication as Patterned Repetition

There are a variety of ways of interpreting the talmudic passage given in the last section.[7] Here is one plausible reconstruction:

The basic problem is one of establishing that a patient's aberrant reaction (head nodding, head shaking) is a meaningful action that should be given legal effect. The examination involves asking questions of a yes/no type, to ensure that the voiceless person is responding appropriately. Thus far does the Mishna establish. Its commentary, the Gemara, points out several problems that arise, and their suggested resolution. The difficulties relate to problems in the structure as well as content of communication; the resolutions, to the format of the examination and its content.

The passage seems reminiscent of a scientific experiment, to answer the question: Is the husband intentionally communicating through head movement? The reliability of the study is established through replication: The test is done three times. The experimenter wishes to control for, or to eliminate, confounding variables, such as intermittent tremor, and so manipulates the experimental design in terms of timing and variation of appropriate response.[8]

We can, perhaps, go even further than that, to describe the kind of experiment being conducted. Consider the problem of establishing communication with an alien species. The message sent must perform two tasks: First, it must be evident that the message is not a natural phenomenon, but rather emanates from an intelligent life form intending to communicate. Second, the message must be decodable, that is, it must point to or explain a language understood in common by the party sending, and that receiving, the message. We could further suppose, to keep this example parallel to the case of the person rendered speechless, that a binary format to the message—yes/no, head-nod/head-shake—is the limit of the medium of communication.

Communication, whatever its form, contains two elements: pattern and repetition. To show that the message is meaningful, then, a message of a certain degree of complexity (pattern) must be sent consistently. This is the subject of the first colloquy in the Gemara. The possibility that what appears to be intentional communication is in fact a nonintentional motion of purely physiological causation needs to be addressed: "Let us be concerned that perhaps he suffers a tremble of 'no, no'; or if not, a tremble of 'yes, yes.'" A nod or shake of the head may simply be automatic behavior or symptoms of the patient's underlying disease. The response to that is that he is asked questions "in stages" (serugin; literally, "strips"), which Rashi explains as follows: "We wait an hour after he has nodded to a question, and then we return and ask him the selfsame question again."

That satisfies the need for repetition, but not for patterning; it is possible that this apparent communication is simply an intermittent but recurring natural phenomenon: "Yet we should be concerned that perhaps he has a tremor in stages!" (A similar problem: Extremely regular radio signals, which were at first thought by a few to represent an alien civilization's efforts at communication, were found later to have in fact been the result of a previously unknown astronomical phenomenon, pulsars.) The element of patterning is supplied by asking a series of questions that should yield staggered, alternating responses, "no-yes-yes-no-no-yes": "We ask him one question of No, and two of Yes, and two of No, and one of Yes."

We have now demonstrated, through patterned repetition, that the phenomenon observed is meaningful. However, for it to constitute communication it needs to be decodable into a language understood in common by both parties. (And, as was argued earlier, competence to consent—to the preparation of a *get* no less than to receiving treatment—requires communication.) In interstellar communication, this may be attempted by using mathematical sequences or physical constants that should be common to the experience of both parties. This is the contribution of the school of Rabbi Yishmael: "They speak to him of summer matters during winter [the rainy season], and of winter matters during summer."

Competence and Mutual Comprehension

Once again, there is a problem: The experience of two races may be dissimilar, in unsuspected ways, leading to a breakdown in the decodability of the message. A proposal to use representations of carbon compounds, as a surrogate representation of organic life, will misfire if directed toward a silicate-based life-form. In the same way, here, the experience of the speechless husband may cause what seems to others to be a nonsensical message: He asks to be covered in blankets in August because he feels a chill. Therefore, a lowest common denominator of language is sought, in this case, relating to consumption within a local refrigerator-free agrarian society. The yes/no questions relate to seasonal fruit: "Could I get you a peach now, if you wanted one?" is a yes question in the summer, a no question in the winter.

It is somewhat unclear how many questions are asked, and how often, from the talmudic discussion given here; it is hard to tell whether some comments add to the previous suggestion or supplant it. A conservative reading would have it that the Gemara requires six correct answers to questions (no-yes-yes-no-no-yes), with the same results following an hour's delay (in accord with Rashi's view), to constitute one examination of communication. However, the examination itself, as the Mishna states, needs to be repeated three times. The reason? In Judaism, a legal presumption—in this case, that the person's actions are intended as meaningful communication—must be grounded in threefold repetition. To return to our analogy with a scientific experiment, finally, we could point out that the odds that a person whose responses are random rather than meaningfully responsive would successfully complete this examination are less than one chance in a hundred billion ($\frac{1}{2}$ to the 36th power).[9]

The same principles apply, of course, today. Some patients with profound paralysis retain the ability to communicate solely through blinking. With them, the first task is to ensure that their blinking is meaningful, and similar forms of patterned repetition in yes/no questions are employed to this end. The second task, ensuring a common language, is tested when we examine to see whether a patient remains oriented to time, place, and person. (If you like, we might say that the school of Rabbi Yishmael had introduced a protocol for testing orientation to time.)

It is therefore instructive to compare one standard psychological protocol for assessing impaired patients, the Western Aphasia Battery.[10] The first step to assessing the patient's understanding of the spoken word (what psychologists choose to call "auditory verbal comprehension") consists of asking a series of yes/no questions. Just as in the Talmud, the series is designed so that the correct responses are staggered. (In this battery of twenty questions, the correct answers start: no, no, yes, no, yes, no, yes . . .)

The kind of comprehension being tested yields an interesting comparison as well. The first nine of these questions test the patient's self-orientation—for example, Is your name Smith? Are you a man? The next five test the patient's understanding of present circumstances—for example, Are you wearing red pajamas? Are we in a hotel? There is no parallel to these kinds of questions in the Talmud, because, I believe, the minimal mental abilities for which these questions test are not relevant to whether the person is competent to exercise a legal choice such as divorce.

The last set of six questions tests orientation to general facts outside of the immediate situation. It is interesting to note that of this set of six, two questions relate to the weather and seasons (Does it snow in July? Does March come before June?), and a third question to fruits (Do you eat a banana before you peel it?)![11]

The Minima of Competence and the Problem of Competence

Granting, as a theoretical matter, that this reflects three minimal conditions for competency—communication, choice, common language—will not, of course, resolve all the practical questions that testing competency raises. To a degree, in fact, it fosters them. A patient is told the electrodes being attached are for an electrocardiogram, and says no more: Has she expressed a choice, refusal of the EKG, or general disgust at how many of her body functions are failing and hope that her heart at least is stable? A patient, deeply demented, is told by a nurse to speak up if it hurts when he is turned; he is turned, and moans softly. Is he saying that it hurts, expressing hurt as a nonintentional automatic response, or . . . ?

The hospital milieu is particularly fraught with the potential for disagreement on these matters. Family members of stroke patients often report responsiveness when none is observed by the neurological or nursing staff. Sometimes, this may be a function of the time spent by the family members with the patient, giving them the opportunity to observe rare lucid and reactive periods. Often, it represents self-deception, a triumph of hope over observation. Also, when a patient is intermittently or marginally responsive, there is a strong tendency on the part of many to overinterpret the patient's responses, particularly those given to very leading, tendentious questions ("You still want to live, don't you?").

I do not mean to minimize the importance and difficulties of these practical concerns. However, we could not begin to address them before getting clear about the underlying theoretic of competency.

Competence and Roles: Competence as Capability and as Authorization

The last section described some necessary conditions for competency: common language, communication, choice. These conditions are not, together, sufficient for competency, nor, indeed, could they have been. We have not yet supplied a specification—competent for what? For it is impossible to define competency in the abstract.

Forms of Competency and Their Components: Example One—Chess

It is usual, in the common law, to describe a variety of forms of competency: to prepare a will, to marry, to commercially contract, to stand trial, to consent to treatment, and so forth. The associated standard for each of these differs from those of the others, so that the common law assigns competence as a sectoral rather than global matter. Those who write of fully individuated—or decisional, or situational—competence could most charitably be understood as suggesting that the application of a sectoral standard may yield varying results within the sector in question, depending upon the choice at hand.

In each case, the x for which one's competency is judged represents action in fulfillment of some social role, and the significance associated with one's being "competent to x" is that one's $x$ing is as a result legally effective. An ascription of competency, that is, includes a claim about facts as well as about values: The person has the ability to fulfill the role in question (fact), and the person's actions in this role should be morally and legally acknowledged (values). I will deal with competency as a juncture of these two claims: The person in question must be *found* (fact) to have the capability to x, and the courts or some other organ of society must *decide* (values) that the person is authorized to x.

Much confusion may result from a failure on the part of analysts to keep these two components distinct. To see this, consider a kind of social role without the charged legal implications of the categories here: chess playing. When we say that someone is able to play chess, we could simply mean that he or she knows how to move the pieces and is familiar with the rules of the game. This person, that is, is capable of playing chess.

The capability to play chess represents an absolute precondition to chess playing. Lacking capability, whatever else a person might be doing—playing a different game, arranging the pieces artistically, etc.—he is not playing chess. It is also, in general, a threshold quality. A person either does or does not know the rules of the game.[12]

Authorization, however, is a much less defined, much more variable, component of competency to fulfill some social role. Authorization will, given liberal and meritocratic leanings, focus most clearly upon the attainment of some level of skill, over and above bare capability; and the level or threshold of skill that may be required for fulfilling some social role depends upon the nature and purpose of the role in question. A chess club run in a community center may require nothing more than capability to play chess, a group for "serious" players may impose more strenuous requirements, tournaments on a national level still more, and so forth. Social purposes will control the choice of the requisite level of skill. The chess club may want to attract people to the game, to introduce as many people as possible to chess. The more serious group has members who want to hone their skills against challenging players. The organizers of the tournament have money and prestige at stake; they don't want to disappoint their fans.

Authorization, unlike capability, is negotiable and, perhaps for that very reason, debatable. In addition, the definition of authorization (like the definition of a level of skill) is vulnerable to non-chess considerations, including social values. A parent may not allow a son to play penny-ante chess in the park until the child has demonstrated both some skill in the game and the common sense not to get in over his head. A neighborhood chess freelancer will have different values in mind in choosing a mark. The theme in choosing the level of skill necessary for authorization may be an associated risk-benefit calculation on the part of the person choosing. The parent asks whether it is safe to allow the son to play chess in that setting, as does the chess freelancer—with very different ends in view and, perhaps, correspondingly different results.

Capability and Authorization:
Example Two—Competency of Criminal Defendants

The same kind of distinctions and resulting points may be observed in considering legal issues of competency. Consider a couple of examples drawn from the criminal law. For a criminal defendant to be competent to stand trial, the defendant must have the mental capacity to understand the nature and gravity of the charges he faces and also be capable of consulting with his attorney in the preparation of a defense to those charges. These are distinct. Just as a patient may be able to understand the nature of a treatment recommendation but be unable to participate in decision making (because of an inability to communicate, as was true of the locked-in patient, Ms. M, or an inability to decide, as was true of Ms. V), so a defendant may understand the nature of the charges but be unable to meaningfully communicate with an attorney.

On one level, this may be taken as an elementary requirement of fairness: What is the point of holding a trial if the defendant is unable to meaningfully participate? But there are answers—more or less convincing—that may be offered to that challenge. On another level, however, we may understand these components of competency to stand trial as flowing from the definition of the social role of defendant. In the "criminal trial game" as it is played in North America, at any rate, the defendant is called upon to play a social role. A person who cannot be made to understand the nature and gravity of the charges against him is like a person who does not know he is playing chess; one who cannot consult with his attorney, like one who cannot move the chess pieces.

These speak solely to capability, which in this case suffices to establish authorization. Certainly defendants vary in (for example) the skill with which they can play the criminal trial game, but society has no real concern that only those defendants who know how to play the system well can play. Rather, our trial system establishes a non-negotiable minimum for a defendant to be capable of playing the role assigned in the elements of competence to stand trial.

As another example, take competency to undergo the death penalty. Consider this case: A person has been found guilty of murder and sentenced to death. The trial, let it be granted, was fair. This implies, among other things, that the defendant was competent to stand trial and was legally responsible at the time he committed the crime. In the course of time, however, this defendant has lapsed into insanity. He appears at this time unable to comprehend that he is currently legally incarcerated, nor that the state is about to take his life, having found him guilty of having committed murder. (In his schizophrenic fugue, he believes that he has been captured by a demonic cult that is planning to kill him to prevent him from revealing the secret conspiracy he has unearthed.) The United States Supreme Court has ruled that in such a case, he is incompetent to be executed. Again, what is in question is capability: To be jailed is not the same as to be kidnapped, to be executed by the state is not the same as to be killed by a demonic cult, and a person who cannot grasp these distinctions and how they apply to his own situation is not capable of playing the social role of the capital offender.[13]

Social Policy and Variable Conceptions of Competency

In these cases, as was noted, only capability is in question; no social policy calls for the defendant or convict to demonstrate any particular skill or other prerequisite in order to be authorized to play the role in question. Now consider competency to perform transactions on the futures market in commodities, as compared with competency to prepare a will (competency for testation). In both cases, similar mental capacities are engaged regarding the person's awareness of his or her financial assets. (In the case of wills, a further mental capacity—awareness of one's personal and family situation—is required as well.)[14] A person who, by reason of mental aberration, has a completely mistaken view of the extent of his or her property is incompetent in either case, and a court may intervene and nullify the transaction on that basis. But what if mental illness has left the transactor marginally competent; what if the person has a partial grasp of these matters, for example, a very general sense of his holdings? The courts, as a matter of policy—to avoid the potentially endless litigation that wills can engender—have held more lenient views concerning competency to prepare a will than competency to engage in financial speculation.[15] The strong social interest in the secure and peaceful transfer of property after death causes courts to demand less skill of the testator than of the financial speculator, even if the complexity of the two transactions in question is similar.

Traditionally, a similar consideration stood at the center of contract law. As we saw in the case of Mr. U, incompetency is a double-edged sword. A person whose contracts and agreements are void because of his incompetency is both protected from his own folly and at the same time excluded from the marketplace. Despite a child's legal incompetency, therefore, in early times an exception had been forged on behalf of contracts for food and other necessities of life, so that an incompetent minor not be legally protected to the point of starvation.[16] At the same time, some degree of understanding must be present for the child to have the *capability* to contract. If, for example, the child did not understand that she was handing over money and in return was to receive food, the child lacks the capability to make such a contract, which is an absolute bar to competency—fortunately so, since in such a case the law would not have advanced the child's interests at all by granting the legal power to contract.

By keeping the elements of capability and authorization distinct, we are forced to directly debate any elements of social utility or other values that may enter into a competency determination. This is useful when evaluating a "variable theory of competency" such as that proposed by Drane.

For Drane, a patient is competent to agree to needed medical treatment provided only that the patient is aware of the situation; whereas, to refuse that treatment, the patient would have to provide an intelligible rationale for such refusal. It is arguable whether a person agreeing to needed medical treatment out of a simple "awareness of the situation," without the ability to understand the risks and benefits of the treatment options (a capacity exceeding that which Drane would require for these choices that he favors), has the capability of playing the role of consenting patient. Who is to know what a compliant demented patient was thinking in acquiescing to treatment? Has that person fulfilled the social role of patient or been employed as an unsuspecting actor in a charade performed for the benefit of others?

Less satisfactory are Drane's requirements for competency to refuse unarguably (by whom?) beneficial treatment. Cashing out the meaning of this heightened requirement, Drane writes,

> Persons who are incapable of making the effort required to control destructive behavior (substance abusers and sociopaths), as well as neurotic persons, hysterical persons, and persons who are ambivalent about their choice, would all be incompetent to refuse life-saving treatment.[17]

Such a strict standard of competency obviously goes well beyond capability to consent. Because he has failed to distinguish between the discovery of capability and the decision of authorization, Drane fails to face squarely what social value is served by requiring this enhancement in skill on behalf of authorization. Armed with the distinction, we are in a position to decide whether the value of protection of life stands supreme as a social value or whether it must instead compete with others, such as respect for individual, idiosyncratic choice.

Drane's proposal might be said to be paternalistic, but I would argue that it is bad parenting. Imagine raising a daughter in this way, allowing her to make choices only when the parent judges it's good for her. What will such a child grow up thinking about choice, authority, autonomy? What messages would such a child infer regarding dependency, second-guessing of self and of others, the externalized conscience and responsibility?

The reader's values may, of course, differ from my own, and be more in accord with Drane's. But such a disagreement should in any event be engaged squarely, rather than finessed by smuggling values into a tendentious definition of competency. Drane's requirements of competency go beyond discovering whether a person has capability— they involve deciding whether a capable person's decision should be authorized under particular circumstances. Only when we see that there is here a clear matter of choice, of social policy, may the argument fairly be joined.

To sum up, then: If one is competent to x—with x representing some social role, such as contract maker, defendant, patient, husband, etc.—then prima facie one's actions as an *x* will be given legal effect. To be competent to *x*, one must both be *capable* of *x*ing and be *authorized* to *x*. For example, one might need to be sufficiently skilled at *x*ing that society deems it reasonable to permit one to *x* (with the legal consequences that ensue). Capability is a non-negotiable requirement, but the degree of skill or other variable required for authorization has been adjusted downward to serve social purposes (as in testation and contracts for necessaries).[18] In principle, the same considerations could require an upward adjustment of skill as well, as in the case of certain discretionary sales or non-necessitous transactions. For example, it has been claimed that in Quebec law greater mental capacity is required to consent to participation in medical research than to consent to treatment.[19]

Social Policy and Competency for Commercial Transactions: Jewish Sources

The distinction between capability and authorization, and the ways in which the requisite degree of skill may be adjusted upward or downward in accordance with social policy, help clarify Jewish views on children's competency to contract for goods and services. Legal majority is reached in Judaism at the ages of twelve (for girls) and thirteen (for boys), provided the child has begun the physical process of puberty. Prior to that age, can a child be deemed competent with respect to commercial transactions? The major talmudic source states:

> As to children: Their purchase is a purchase, and their sale is a sale, in the case of movable property.
> —From when?
> ——R Yehuda would show his son R Yitzchak: As of a child of six or seven.
> ——R Kahana said: As of a child of seven or eight.
> ——We learned in another source *[braita]:* As of nine or ten.
> ——Nor do they disagree, for each case is judged according to his discernment.

—What is the reason?

——R Aba bar Yaakov said in the name of R Yochanan, On behalf of survival's necessities.[20]

Two points bear brief comment:

1. In Judaism, as in many other legal systems, the special economic role played by real estate (as the grounding of wealth, and especially the repository of a family's inheritance down through the generations) results in the imposition of a more formal legal approach than is true for moveable property. Under the civil law of Quebec, to take one example, although an emancipated minor (for example, by reason of marriage) is capable unassisted of simple financial transactions,[21] any of his real estate transactions require court approval.[22]

2. Each of the opinions is expressed as a range of two years (six or seven, seven or eight, nine or ten), rather than as a single cutoff date. This may simply reflect a desire to avoid being too exact in setting down general guidelines regarding matters that are highly individual ("each case is judged according to his discernment"). Alternatively, the paired ages may reflect a Jewish belief that female children mature one year sooner than males, the reason why a female reaches majority at age twelve and a male not until thirteen. By this reading, then, to take one example, R Yehuda would be saying that a child's purchase of moveable property may be valid at age six (if a girl) or age seven (if a boy).

The Talmud's terse and somewhat allusive discussion is expanded upon in Rambam's Code:

A child until the age of six years: His trade with others is invalid. And from six years until he achieves majority: If he understands the nature of commercial transactions *[yodei'a b'tiv masa umatan]*, his purchases and sales are valid, . . . and his gifts endure, whether great or small, whether a gift given while healthy or while moribund. And this matter is by decree of the Sages, as we explained, so that he should not be bereft [yi-batel], and not find anyone to buy from him or sell to him. . . .

All this applies to moveable property, but regarding real estate, he cannot sell or gift until majority. In which case does this law apply? For a child who has no legal guardian, but if he had a legal guardian his acts are invalid. . . .

We examine the child to see if he understands the nature of commercial transactions or not; for one child is wise, understanding and knowledgeable at seven, and another doesn't understand the nature of commercial transactions even at thirteen years.[23]

It seems reasonable to construe the points made here as parallel to the points made earlier. Just as public policy had led the common law to a generous reading of competency (adjusting the required level of skill down) on behalf of contracts for food and other necessaries of life, so too in Jewish sources competency to contract is stretched so that a child is permitted to contract on behalf of the needs of survival. That this is the reason for the enactment is clear from the talmudic passage "What is the reason? R Aba bar Yaakov said in the name of R Yochanan, On behalf of survival's necessities." Rambam and others understand that while this is the reason for taking a lenient approach to children's competence to contract, the enactment's force is not limited to transactions for food and other bare necessities; R Hai Ga'on had earlier in fact restricted the enactment in just this way.

There remains, however, a non-negotiable minimum element to competence to contract, and that is capability. To play the game of commerce, one needs to understand, for example, that after the bargain has been made and the other party has filled his or her end, you are required to fill your own. The basic capability to engage in commerce is expressed well in Rambam's phrase "understands the nature of commercial transactions."

Jewish law supplies instances of adjusting competency upward as well. A person upon reaching the age of majority should be presumed competent in all matters. However, by rabbinic decree, it is required that a thirteen-year-old demonstrate familiarity with commercial transactions before he is permitted to engage in the sale or purchase of real estate. For one who has just achieved majority, that is, the capability to engage in real estate is not presumed but must be demonstrated. And there is one further level imposed: Even after reaching the age of majority and demonstrating capability to trade in real estate, a person is not permitted to sell or gift real estate received in an inheritance from the father or any other person (or given as a deathbed gift) until passing the age of twenty.[24] (These provisions are reminiscent of the variety of encumbrances that may be imposed by a testator upon an estate until the heir has demonstrated certain marks of maturity.)

Jewish Law on Social Policy and Competency to Be Divorced

The distinction between the elements of capability and authorization may be of help in studying another area of competency in Jewish divorce law: that of a wife to be divorced. Because there is an asymmetry in Jewish divorce law—only the husband may initiate divorce proceedings (although, as we have seen in an earlier chapter, the court may force him to do so)—there is a corresponding asymmetry in competency to divorce. A husband must be competent to prepare the *get*, the bill of divorcement; the competency of the wife is to receive a divorce.[25]

The classical sources on this problem are again talmudic, found in the Jerusalem and Babylonian tractates of *Y'vamot*:

A woman who has become a *shota* [a madwoman; the feminine form of *shote*] cannot be sent away. In the school of R Yanai they said, Because of returning *[g'dera, g'rera]*; R Zeira and R Ila both said, Because she cannot guard her *get* [bill of divorce].[26]

R Yitzchak said: As a matter of Torah law a *shota* may be divorced, since she may be sent out against her will. And why did the sages say she may not be divorced? So that she not be treated as ownerless.

—How is this possible? If we were to say that she knows

how to guard her *get* and how to guard herself, how would she be treated as ownerless? And if, instead, she does not know how to guard either herself or her *get,* can she indeed be divorced by Torah law?! Inasmuch as the school of R Yannai had taught, "And he gave it to her hand": She who has a hand to divorce herself, excluding she who has no hand to divorce herself! And the school of R Yishmael had taught, "And he sent her from his house"—one who can be sent away and doesn't return, excluding one who is sent away and returns![27]

    —His [R Yitzchak's] view is only needed as follows: She knows how to guard her get but not her self. As a matter of Torah law she can be divorced, because she knows how to guard her get, but the Sages decided not to have her sent out, so that she not be treated as ownerless.[28]

It should come as no surprise to learn that these short passages and the subsequent efforts to codify them have generated an enormous amount of discussion and disagreement.[29] In a humorous understatement, R Naftali Tzvi Yehuda Berlin, asked to respond to the case of a certain woman, described as clearly capable of guarding her *get* but at times bewildered and confused by various hallucinations, begins his remarks by saying, "His eminence did not explain in what way it is obvious that she knows how to guard her get, insofar as this is not clear in Rambam who had sealed his words regarding a *shote* and did not explain this."[30] The following is one attempt at rationally reconstructing the debate that relies upon the distinction between capability and authorization.

Consider, first, the problem of defining capability for marriage and divorce. Depending upon the social expectations attached to that role, a person entering into marriage may be agreeing to indefinitely long arrangements regarding financial obligations to the spouse, openness to and exclusivity in sexual relations and/or the exercise of reproductive capacity, a commitment to live with the other, or a variety of other matters. (The present difficulty in defining precisely which elements are essential to a marriage is testimony to the nebulous quality the role of spouse has recently acquired.)

Imagine a case in which a wealthy elderly man had married a young woman who in quite short order inherited the whole of his estate. The relatives claim the man, suffering from dementia, had been incompetent to marry, and offer as evidence the fact that the man, dining out with a friend during his honeymoon, appeared not to recognize his bride. "Hello," he had told her when she appeared at their table, with the Old World manners that had been his all his life. "Do I know you? Won't you join me and my friend for dinner?" The capability to marry, to play the game of spouse, implies some mental capacity underlying the commitment to be wed, and whatever these mental capacities might be—people today obviously disagree about this—they seemed to be lacking in this case.

The brief passage from the Jerusalem Talmud appears to express just such a disagreement regarding capability to be divorced. The first view states that the reason that a *shota* cannot be divorced is because of "returning." This puzzling statement can be understood by a cross-reference to the passage in the Babylonian Talmud. The biblical verse had stated that after preparing the bill of divorcement, the husband had put it into his wife's hand. This is understood by the school of R Yanai to mean that she had the capability to accept a *get;* she had—in both senses—grasped what had happened to her. The school of R Yishmael, in support of this explanation, notes that the verse goes on to say that with the acceptance of the *get* the wife has been ejected from her husband's house. It follows then that if a woman, by reason of her mental illness *(shtut),* is incapable of understanding that she no longer lives with her husband—"one who is sent away and returns"—she is thereby incapable of playing the role of divorcee. (Note Rabbenu Asher, who argues that the statements of the two schools are complementary rather than contradictory.)

For this view, basic to the idea of being married is coming together to live with your spouse. Divorce is seen as the negation of marriage, a necessary parting of the ways of spouses. The same definition is one of two suggested derivations for the term divorce—*divortium*—by the Roman jurist Gaius: Those who dissolve their marriage go different ways.[31] A similar kind of socially defined insanity is described by Turnbull in his anthropological work on the Ik, a tribe that had been brutally resettled and, as a result, had suffered a total breakdown in traditional social and family norms. Families of this destitute tribe would expel their children at the age of three, to fend for themselves, to live or to die. Turnbull describes one child who could not grasp that his parents did not love him, would no longer take care of him. His parents explained that the child was insane, "because of returning": The child would creep back to the family home as though he belonged, as though he had never been expelled.[32]

The contrasting view of capability to be divorced in the Jerusalem Talmud (repeated in the Babylonian Talmud and subsequently codified)[33] is that of the ability to "guard her *get.*" In this case, divorce is treated as the assignment of a new legal role rather than the negation of the previous role of "married." The new legal role is expressed in the *get,* and its dominant aspect is the divorced woman's entitlement to the funds earlier promised her in the marriage contract. A woman who is capable of guarding her *get,* therefore, is a person with the mental capacity to recognize her entitlements resulting from divorce and who can seek legal enforcement of the *get.*[34]

In our time, the expression "guarding the *get*" may seem a fanciful and indirect way of speaking about a form of capacity for contract. In talmudic times, however, it conjured up a vivid visual image that may have been completely apt for the kind of capacity for legal self-protection to which the phrase refers. It was a time of social upheaval, of foreign occupation and exile, during which a woman's sole economic prospects may have depended upon her capacity to guard pieces of parchment—her wedding contract and bill of divorcement—and bring them to the attention of the authorities. A wonderful example of a woman who knew well how to guard her *get* was unearthed in the archeological discovery of the Dead Sea Scrolls:

> The largest cache of documents found in the Cave of Letters was the archive of Babata, daughter of Shimeon son of Menahem. Thanks to this woman—who managed to survive two husbands and must have spent most of her life in litigation, either suing the guardians of her fatherless son or being sued

by the various members of her deceased husbands' families—
we have come by a priceless source for the period just preced-
ing the war of Bar-Kokhba. It is full of legal, historical,
geographical and linguistic data. Babata's habit—typical of
many even in our days—of never discarding any slip of paper
in her possession, and her meticulous and orderly nature, are
responsible for the fact that all her documents, thirty-five in
number, were found neatly packed and "filed" by subject-
matter. . . .

Another well-guarded and specially wrapped document
turned out to be Babata's Kethuba [the source's translitera-
tion] (marriage contract). . . . [T]he sum of money she was
given by her husband was "a hundred Tyrians," which according to Jewish law was the sum paid to a widow or a divorcee. . . .

[The document stipulates,] "If I go to my last resting
place before you, you shall dwell in my house and receive
maintenance from it and from my possessions, until such time
as my heirs choose to pay you your Kethuba money."[35]

These are, then, two different views of what it means to be capable of being divorced: the ability to recognize the loss of a previous social role, that of living together with the husband ("because of
returning"), and the ability to recognize the assumption of a new social role, divorcee, with attendant prerogatives ("guard her *get*"). For
the proponents of either view, it represents a non-negotiable minimum: The wife must be capable of being divorced, by Torah law, for
the divorce to take effect.[36]

There remains, however, the question of whether bare capability
to be divorced suffices for authorization. Unanimous opinion rejects
this view. Even when a woman is capable of guarding her *get,* the rabbis enacted a further requirement: She must also be capable of guarding *herself.* The reason given in the Talmud is "so that she not be
treated as ownerless property *[hefker].*" In what sense? This is understood by most commentators as a concern that this *shota,* bereft of a

husband or other male protector, would be prey to rape and sexual assault. (Even were she to "consent" to intercourse, it would remain assault since she lacks the competence to validly consent.)[37] This need not be the full extent of the requirement, however.[38] It is possible to take "guarding her self" as a reference to a more global capacity, the ability to function within society without a husband as a protector.

The threat that the incompetent would be taken as easy sexual prey was in talmudic times very real. We should not congratulate ourselves unduly at having evolved beyond these problems, as recurrent revelations of sexual abuse in orphanages should teach us. But there are other threats, new dangers posed to the mentally infirm, that were unimagined in talmudic times. These too should factor into a decision that a person is in need of, and hence entitled to, protection.

Summing Up: The Talmudic Approach to Capability and Authorization

This requirement that a person be capable of functioning within social expectations is similar to the construct many clinicians have in mind in judging a mental patient's competency. As in the clinical construct, the ability to guard the self is a relative concept, better/worse: In both cases the motivation underlying the construct is a concern for the well-being of the person in question. To take the parallel one step further: The talmudic views of capability to be divorced share several of the characteristics noted earlier regarding our legal system's approach to defining competency, for example, as a binary quality.

The great advantages to the talmudic approach, however, rest in these recognitions: that there are two distinct aspects to competency determinations, the discovery of capability and the decision to grant authorization; that whereas capability is a non-negotiable quality, relating to the ability to grasp the rules of the game in question, authorization may depend upon a particular level of skill or other factors required by broad considerations of social policy and reality; and that both capability and authorization should be given their due, rather than struggle against one another, as is often true of our current legal and clinical approaches.[39]

Defining Mental Illness Within a Social Context: The Need for Protection

A Case Study

As is true of competency, mental illness itself forces society to confront questions of fact and of value: What is it? How is it distinguished from other aspects of the human condition? What does society do about it? These questions were all implicated in the following consultation.

ETHICS DISCUSSION: WORKING THE BORDERLINE

I was invited to participate in a session at the Institute for Family and Community Psychiatry. Dr. P was presenting a case and associated issue with interesting ethical aspects, and he asked me to join in on the common discussion.

Mr. Q is a forty-year-old man with a ten-year psychiatric history at the hospital. He stopped school at grade seven; for the last several years he has been unemployed. His repeated encounters with the hospital have a depressing sameness, e.g.:

- 1983: Diagnosed as having an unspecified personality disorder, later amended to "passive dependent personality disorder." He spent six days at that time in the day hospital. Feeling his only problems were situational, and particularly monetary, he refused medication and was discharged.
- 1984: He came in in crisis, described as an "itinerant male," possibly schizotypic personality disorder, alternatively borderline or antisocial personality disorder, rule out bipolar and schizophrenia. The crisis: He had come to emergency psychiatry desperate at having run out of money.

The pattern recurs over the years. In October, the man approached Dr. P asking for a letter stating that he cannot work because of his psychiatric condition, something that will help him with his welfare check. The issue was whether Dr. P should provide that letter or not, something he was disinclined to do. Dr. F, by contrast, saw no problem in this at all and thought that of course the letter should be provided.

The disagreement between Drs. P and F seemed to be stronger than it needed to be, predicated in part upon a failure to appreciate the new rules with respect to psychiatric disability and welfare. Welfare has all kinds of categories for those available and unavailable to work. The basic issue for this patient is that he will get $622 a month with the letter, $570 without it. The form to be attached to the letter, however, only allows for limited diagnoses grounding assignment to the higher payment, and this patient falls into none of the categories in any obvious way. (The acceptable encodings for psychiatric difficulties include intellectual deficit, coma, epilepsy, anxiety, depression, phobias.) With the letter, the higher payment is automatic. Without it, there is an appeal possible to a committee, including persons from medicine, social work, etc., who decide whether the patient is entitled to the higher bursary.

Dr. P feels that all chronically unemployed persons will have some axis 2 [personality disorder] diagnosis, according to the categories adopted by the psychiatrist's "bible," the American Psychiatric Association's third revised edition of the Diagnostic and Statistical Manual of Mental Disorders (DSM-IIIR). Signing on their behalf would therefore represent the medicalization of a social condition. Dr. F feels that personality disorders are an acceptable form of illness, and should be treated as such. (And Dr. P agrees that personality disorder is a genuine, not artifactual, diagnosis.)

Among the many questions that could be raised in this case are: the genuineness of this diagnosis, and the standard problems associated with psychiatry and the definition of illness/disease/malady etc.; truth and consequences in a world not always truthful and commonly unjust; the ethics of manipulation by patients; the effect of different choices on the physician-patient relationship; and the consequences of medicalizing judgments. In a lengthy discussion, many of these issues were touched upon, and none was brought to ground. Many axes were ground that day, not just DSM-IIIR axes.

I (and I think others) were left in the end somewhat unsure as to what "the" question was here, let alone the answer. The administrative regimen set up by the province appears to allow for—indeed to expect and perhaps even to require—that these borderline cases (in both senses of the term) be dealt with by the appeals committee. At various times both Drs. P and F, as well as others, agreed that the committee is structurally better suited to be a decision maker on this issue of intermingled medical and social judgments than the individual treating psychiatrist. So much confusion about the administrative arrangements—how appeals are lodged, what exactly the form requires, what the form's categories encompass, etc.—was expressed at the meeting that no clear conclusion was possible.

Dr. P raised what to me remains the most intriguing point: the idea that all chronically unemployed persons would have a diagnosis of personality disorder. The canons of jurisprudence and legal interpretation require us to read the regulations in a charitable way, that is, to interpret them when ambiguous so that they make sense. In that setting, his view that personality disorder is not per se an eligibility condition must be granted. The obvious intention in segmenting the population on welfare was to differentiate (by need, merit, or otherwise). Including one route to a higher monthly welfare check via psychiatric diagnosis was intended to differentiate within the broader class of the unemployed. This differentiating purpose is pragmatically inconsistent with an interpretation of psychiatric diagnosis that allows all of the unemployed into what was supposed to be a limited, privileged category.

As this example illustrates, the problems of how to assign a social role to a person suffering mental illness are not reducible to the question of the definition of mental illness itself. In this case, both discussants agreed that borderline personality disorder represented a bona fide diagnosis and, indeed, an acceptable basis for psychiatric intervention and treatment. (As a matter of fact, Dr. P's practice is very largely composed of persons suffering from this disorder.) The same is true of another major issue posed by mental illness, namely, forcible confinement and medical and psychiatric intervention. In most jurisdictions, certainly within North America, the fact of a patient's mental illness does not settle the question of forcible confinement, but only introduces it. The patient in question must be a demonstrable danger to himself/herself or others, as a result of the mental illness in question.

I will not deal, except incidentally, with the difficult philosophical and conceptual problems posed by the definition of mental illness itself, but rather will concentrate on the issue of social reaction to mental illness, through involuntary confinement and treatment, competency determinations and otherwise. In Judaism too, I believe, the emphasis in discussing mental illness was placed not upon its definition—a matter treated as self-evident from disordered thought, speech, and behavior—but upon the extent to which its presence places the *shote* at risk.

The Talmudic Definition of Mental Illness and Physicalist Views

The *locus classicus* for all Jewish normative discussions of mental illness is found in a passage from the tractate *Chagiga* of the Babylonian Talmud:

> Mishna: All are required to appear [at the Temple during the three major festivals, Passover, Pentecost, and Sukkot], except for the deaf-mute, the *shote,* and the minor.[40]
>
> Gemara: Our rabbis learned: Who is a *shote*? [Rashi: The one spoken of generally, who is exempt from commandments and from punishments, and whose purchase is no purchase, and whose sale is no sale.] One who goes out alone at night, and one who sleeps in graveyards, and one who tears his garments.
>
> —It was taught: Rav Huna said: [One is not considered a madman] until he does all of them together; R Yochanan said: Even one of them.

——How are we to understand this? If the case is one in
which he did it in a mad fashion, even one suffices; if the
case is one in which he did not do it in a mad fashion,
even all of them will not.

——Rather: He did it in a mad fashion, but: one who sleeps in
a graveyard—let us say that he did that so that a spirit of
impurity will dwell upon him [Rashi: A demonic spirit
which will assist him to be a sorcerer]; one who goes out
alone at night—let us say that he was seized by [the illness]
gandripas; and one who tears his garments—let us say he
is preoccupied. Once he has done them all, he is like [an
ox] who has wounded an ox and a donkey and a camel,
and has a presumption of viciousness *[mu'ad]* for all.

—Rav Papa said: Had Rav Huna heard that which was
taught, "Who is a madman? One who loses everything [or,
destroys everything; *me'abed kol ma shenotnim lo*] given to
him," he would have reversed himself.

——They asked him: He would have reversed himself regarding one who tears his garments, for this is similar, or
would he rather have reversed himself regarding all?—
The answer is undecided *[Taiku].*[41]

The Babylonian passage provides what seems to be a behavioral
triad of symptoms: going out alone at night, sleeping in graveyards,
tearing one's clothes. (To these the Jerusalem Talmud[42] adds a fourth
symptom, alluded to here: "losing all given to him.") It is tempting to
read this talmudic passage as though it were trying to provide a description of mental illness—a diagnosis, such as a psychiatrist of our
times might provide—and to try to tie this description to contemporary diagnostic nomenclature. R Avraham Dov Levin,[43] following earlier sources,[44] identifies going out alone at night and sleeping in
graveyards with an excess of *hamarah hashchorah,* tearing garments
with excessive *hamarah halvanah* or *hamarah ha'adumah,* and losing
all he is given with mental retardation.

Levin's proposal illustrates what is wrong with this physicalist approach. (The concept of a physicalist approach was brought up in my

Introduction.) What is *hamarah hashchorah*? A term appearing with some frequency in post-talmudic rabbinic literature, it is commonly identified with melancholia (often *malankuniya* in this literature).[45] *Hamarah hashchorah,* which could mean, literally, "black bitterness," may equally or more likely mean "black bile."[46] Its association with melancholia appears to represent a clear codification of the then-current humoral theory of disease, according to which depression is caused by the humoral imbalance of excessive black bile.[47]

Diagnosis implies an underlying theory of disease and causation, and a particular diagnosis only makes sense on behalf of those who share the underlying theory presumed by the diagnostic system. Were we to understand the talmudic passage as listing a diagnosis or diagnoses, therefore, its import would be restricted to those sharing the talmudic theory of mental illness. (Without entering into that latter question, I will note that those rabbinic authors that are attempting to remain true to the talmudic theory by adopting the traditional humoral theory of disease, a theory rife among the post-talmudic rabbinic authorities, particularly the Rishonim, must inevitably fail, inasmuch as there are no clear references to a humoral theory in the literature of the talmudic period.)

There are two alternatives to reading the passage as diagnosis. It may be describing instead *symptoms* of mental illness; alternatively, by the common talmudic method that uses concrete examples, by alluding to some characteristics of mental illness. The first of these alternatives implies that the behaviors listed have a unique status, that only to those persons exhibiting these behaviors may the rabbinic concept of *shote* be imputed.[48] And support for the view that these symptoms were considered pathognomonic of mental illness may be found in the fact that the triad reappears, interestingly, in the New Testament story of Jesus's encounter with a man possessed by demons, who are caused to depart from the man and to enter the Gadarene herd of swine. The "clinical impression" of this madman is provided in the verse describing his meeting with Jesus: "And as he [Jesus] stepped out on land, there met him a man from the city who had demons; for a long time he had worn no clothes, and he lived not in a house but among the tombs."[49]

But the view that these symptoms are in and of themselves definitive of mental illness must, I think, be rejected, on logical as well as
textual grounds. Logically, what possible basis is there for thinking
that these and only these symptoms bear the severe consequence of
rabbinic incompetence? Commonly, when a seemingly arbitrary set of
conditions is granted special significance in the Talmud, a dogmatic
reason is supplied, such as the fact that the set has been singled out in
Scripture itself as special, explicitly or by inference (see, for example,
the laws of purity and impurity, or the list of forbidden Sabbath activities). Neither the Talmud itself, nor any commentator that I have
found, suggests any such basis for the *Chagiga* triad. (As we will see
later in this chapter, the biblical precedent for mental illness might
suggest a different set of associated symptoms.)

In the absence of any dogmatic reason for singling out the triad,
there must be some natural characteristic that they share that singles
them out for special legal and moral significance; but if that is the
case, then the behaviors listed, rather than being uniquely definitive
of mental illness, must rather be emblematic of some unique characteristic—in other words, our second alternative must be true.

Textually, too, the triad cannot represent symptoms definitive of
mental illness, or the talmudic passage begs the question.[50] After listing the symptoms, the Talmud requires that one or more of them be
done "in a mad fashion," *b'derekh shtut*. If these behaviors are definitive symptoms of mental illness, this requirement of the Talmud
would involve it in a circular definition; it would be saying, "Mad acts
are (defined as) *x*, *y*, and *z*, provided they are done in a mad manner."
To avoid circularity, the listed behaviors must be pointing to something about madness, *shtut*, rather than constituting a definition of
shtut itself.

Maimonides's Rationalistic Approach
to Defining Mental Illness

We are forced, therefore, to the third view: Rather than providing
diagnoses of mental illness or a privileged list of symptoms, the Talmud should be understood as presenting a class of symptoms of madness that share in common some additional important characteristic.

What might that characteristic be? We may infer one theory from Rambam's discussion of insanity:

> The *shote* is interdicted *[pasul]* for testimony by Torah decree for he is not duty-bound by *mitzvot [sheʾeino ben mitzva];* and not merely a madman who goes about naked, and breaks utensils, and throws rocks; rather, anyone who has become mad and whose mind is found to be always confused regarding some matter, even though he can speak and inquire in relevant ways on other matters: He is interdicted, and considered among the class of madmen.
>
> The *nichpe* [probably: epileptic] at the time of his seizure is interdicted, but at the time he is healthy is fit. The same law applies to the one who is *nichpe* at regular intervals as to the one who is always subject to seizures at no set time—this, provided his mind is not always confused; for there are *nichpim* who are mad even when they are healthy. It is necessary to closely examine the testimony of *nichpim.*
>
> 10: Those who are most profoundly intellectually disabled *[peti bʾyoter],* who cannot recognize statements that are mutually contradictory, and do not understand statements as everyone else does, and similarly those in panic or anxiety and those who are most insane, are in the class of *shotim.* This matter is in accord with what the judge shall see, for it is impossible through writing to be precise on this matter.[51]

Rambam may have been the first rabbinic authority to interpret the symptoms in *Chagiga* as an exemplary rather than exhaustive list.[52] What specifically is the defining characteristic of this class of mad behavior? What is the legal definition of mental illness? For Rambam, the major common denominator appears to be cognitive disturbance, what a psychiatrist would call a thought disorder, as opposed to the behavioral or emotional components of mental disorder. For Rambam, the broad class of *shotim* is defined as including "anyone who has become mad and whose mind is found to be always confused regarding some matter"; someone the special class of epileptics is judged competent when not undergoing a seizure, "provided his mind is not always confused," that is, his thoughts are not disordered; the *peti,* a rabbinic category applied to the mentally handicapped, is defined by Rambam in an austere, rationalistic way: those "who cannot recognize statements that are mutually contradictory, and do not understand statements as everyone else does." Central to Rambam's view of legal insanity, then, is irrationality; a miscellany of mental illnesses or symptoms that fail to fit this model—"those in panic or anxiety" and the rather mysterious and unexplained class of "those who are most insane"—are introduced incidentally and are off-handedly assimilated to that legal treatment assigned to and created for the central concept of thought disorder.

I described earlier reasons I consider sufficient to reject two views of the Talmud's discussion in *Chagiga,* viz., that it was describing specific mental illnesses (diagnosis) or that it was defining a set of symptoms that are uniquely significant for legal purposes. I therefore join with Rambam in choosing the third path: The Talmud intended, with the examples it provided, to point to a legally significant quality that may accompany mental illness. Where we part, however, is in identifying that quality. To define mental illness for legal purposes as irrationality is perfectly consistent with the Maimonidean project.[53] It indeed fits Rambam's views far more closely than it does the passage in *Chagiga* with which we began, for the latter is referring to some commonality over and above madness itself.[54] To see this, we need to return to the talmudic discussion for a closer examination, for it appears that while disordered thought is surely characteristic of *shtut,* and perhaps necessary for it, it is not sufficient. Rather, disordered thought needs to be combined with behavior that is aberrant in a particular way.

A Normative Understanding of the Talmudic Definition: Mental Illness as Posing a Danger to Self or to Others

Such disagreement and byplay as exists in *Chagiga* is concerned with whether all elements of the triad are required to establish a person within the legal class of *shote,* as R Huna has it, or only one, in accordance with the view of R Yochanan. There appears, however, to be considerable consensus within the passage, which is worth mining for an underlying view of legally relevant mental illness:

- All agree that the triad (viz., going out alone at night, sleeping in graveyards, tearing clothes) represents paradigmatic signs of mental illness. (Bearing in mind the passage quoted from Luke, it could even be that these three signs had come to constitute a kind of folkloric shorthand for mental illness.)
- A fourth sign, "losing all that is given to him," incontrovertibly belongs to the list as well. It appears in fact to have a special status: The passage discusses the fact that this sign alone may for R Huna be sufficient to establish *shtut*, unlike the other signs, which (in his view) must be done in combination.
- A parallel passage in the Jerusalem Talmud[55] also posits a special status to this fourth sign. It is there suggested by R Abun that R Yochanan's view (that a single sign is sufficient) only refers to "losing all given to him"; as R Abun says there, even a *shote* among *shotim* does not lose all that is given to him.
- All of the signs reflect behavior, and in fact go beyond verbal behavior to action.
- Although all of the behaviors listed are on the surface aberrant, the Talmud recognizes the possibility that each can occur in the absence of *shtut*.

What underlying lessons may be gleaned from these points? Three clues seem present:

- First, the legal attribution of mental illness is centrally concerned with behavior, rather than with disarranged thought or even words, contrary to the Maimonidean view.[56]
- Second, note the alternative explanations for the talmudic signs that rebut the presumption that one acting in this

way is a *shote*. Those alternative explanations (posited in TB *Chagiga;* and, in the case of the fourth sign, "losing all given to him," in TY *T'rumot*) are themselves far from "normal" behavior. The behavior in question, it is said, may be caused by an illness other than *shtut* (going out at night by *gandripas*,[57] losing all given to him by *kordiakos*),[58] by extreme inattentiveness to one's surroundings (tearing garments caused by "preoccupation"),[59] or even by the pursuit of evil ends (sleeping in a graveyard for purposes of consorting with evil spirits).

These alternative explanations point to the talmudic view that the odd, the eccentric, the passing strange, and even the evil—aberrant behaviors, in and of themselves—do not signify mental illness for legal purposes. Something more, or, at any rate, different, is needed.

- Third, whatever opaque characteristic is held in common by the three signs is relatively more transparent in the fourth, losing all that is given to him, a sign with recognized special status in both the Babylonian and Jerusalem passages.

These essential clues are seized upon by the *Chatam Sofer* in an important responsum on the juridical aspects of mental illness:

The *shote* spoken of throughout occurs when he actively performs actions that demonstrate his derangement and his confusion of thought. It is clear in the [passage from the] Jerusalem Talmud that a man whose mind is totally deranged in such a fashion that all of his actions are tainted, who has no understanding to guard his clothes from tearing and to guard himself from going out [at night] and sleeping in a place of danger or to preserve what is given to him [is what is called a *shote*]. . . . One who loses all that is given to him is considered as the uttermost *shote*.[60]

In brief, the common characteristic of these aberrant behaviors is that they reflect the *shote*'s inability to look out for his or her own best interests. Action done in wanton disregard of one's own person or property is the definitive mark of *shtut*. It is for this reason that "losing all that is given him" is singled out as paradigmatic among this set.

Is this a fair common denominator for these behaviors? While it may be clear that losing whatever you are given, or its subset, tearing up your own clothes, reflects reckless disregard of your own property interests, what do the other signs signify? To answer this, we need to begin by imaginatively projecting ourselves into the world that the Talmud reflects. In that world, travel was always dangerous, and travel at night still more so. Traveling alone at night was tantamount to negligent suicide: "One who goes out on the road alone before the rooster's crow: His blood is upon his own head."[61] A similar admonishment is embellished in another talmudic passage:

> Our rabbis learned: Three sounds travel from one end of the earth to the other, and they are these: The sound of the sun's passing; the sound of the hordes of Rome; and the sound of a soul at the moment that it departs from the body. . . . We learned in accordance with R Shila, One who departs upon the road before the rooster's crow, his blood is upon his own head.[62]

[One plausible reading of this passage is as a poetic causal description of the reason one is prohibited from going out alone at night. The reason is connected to the Roman presence: When night goes down ("the sun's passing") Roman bandits emerge ("the sound of the hordes of Rome") to pillage and murder ("the sound of a soul at the moment that it departs").]

A similar stricture is found regarding another sign:

> R Shimon ben Yochai said, Five things there are whose doer bears soul-guilt [i.e., who bears guilt as though he had committed a capital offense] and whose blood is upon his own head: . . . One who sleeps in graveyards so that an unclean

spirit should rest upon him, for occasionally this endangers him.[63]

In fact, in one source the third sign is implicated as well: "Three things there are that remove a person from the world: . . . One who sleeps in graveyards; and some say, even one who tears up his garments in his anger."[64]

To conclude, then: The state of *shtut* is established when a person acts in wanton disregard of his or her own property and well-being. These actions must be done in a manner indicating an underlying mental illness or disorientation of thought ("in a mad fashion"), and alternative possible explanations (e.g., that the action was caused by another illness) may need to be rebutted. *Shtut* is a legal designation, then, based upon a finding that a person's mental illness has led him or her to act in ways dangerous to the self.

This is a close analogue to the legal standard adopted by those many jurisdictions that provide for interdicting persons who are shown to be a danger to themselves or others by reason of mental illness. Here, however, the Western regime of rights and the Jewish regime of duties again come to a parting of the ways. The Western system interdicts the legally insane by restricting their rights, which may include the right to refuse treatment or even the right to freedom of movement. The *shote* in Judaism has his or her social role restricted by losing the capacity to exercise duty—literally, to be *bar-mitzva* (for males) or *bat-mitzva* (for females).

Rambam's language, in the passage quoted earlier, was therefore meant to be understood quite precisely: The reason the *shote* may not validly testify in court, Rambam wrote, is because "he is not duty-bound by *mitzvot [she'eino ben mitzva]*."[65] The category of *shtut* does not mean he has lost the right or privilege of testifying, but rather the duty of testifying; the role of witness in a Jewish court is restricted to those acting under pressure of duty. In precisely the same way, in commenting upon the passage in *Chagiga* that states that those who suffer from *shtut* are not required to appear at the Temple during holidays, Rashi, the premier talmudic scholar, comments, "For they do not possess intelligence *[lav bnei dei'a ninhu]*, and they are exempt from commandments."[66]

Competency, Consent to Treatment, and Other Social Roles

The differences between competency in a regime of rights and of duties returns us to the earlier distinction between competency as capability and as authorization. It was argued that while the elements of capability could be deduced from the activity in question, decisions about authorization rest upon broader social values and understandings. The determination of authorization in practice may, of course, be done well or poorly; ideally, however, it should reflect agreed-upon social interests. The fewer such interests, the lower the standard for determining authorization. But can authorization be dispensed with completely?

Recognizable Reasons: Playing the "Patient Game"

In some earlier work, I had proposed a theory of competency to consent to medical treatment or research in part motivated by that issue.[67] Put in terms of the categories introduced here, the theory ran as follows: From our understanding of what it means to be a patient (or research subject) there follow certain requirements, "rules" of the "patient game." These requirements, which constitute capability to consent, are similar but not identical to those that make up capability to contract. Those capable to consent should not be authorized to do so unless they can provide recognizable reasons for the choices they make.

In our culture, the "patient game," broadly speaking, begins by requiring communication: one party making decisions based upon information supplied by an expert. Treatment could, of course, be provided on another basis, but that is not the way we play the game. An illustrative anecdote: Bismarck, the "Iron Chancellor," summoned a doctor to treat him for a painful foot condition. The doctor came and examined him and then proceeded to ask Bismarck questions toward establishing a medical history. Bismarck, who was conducting affairs of state throughout the examination, told the doctor to spare him the questions and just do something about the foot. The doctor began to pack his bags and take his leave, and Bismarck asked him what was wrong. The doctor replied that he, as a physician, was accustomed to speaking to his patients in establishing a diagnosis. A person who wants to be treated without being asked or answering questions does not wish to be treated by a physician, but rather by a veterinarian. Veterinarians are accustomed to treating their patients without speaking to them.[68] A certain disposition and capability are therefore involved: To be a patient requires something more than being a sick mammal.

This communication involves not simply form but content: It needs to be effectively directed toward elucidating a choice of medical treatment. From this follows the common view that a patient's competency to consent to a particular treatment requires that the patient understand and appreciate the nature of the treatment recommended and that of any alternatives to this treatment, as well as their associated risks and benefits. (To choose a medical treatment requires something more than blindly picking out one card from the deck.) We may also add a factor spoken of earlier, but rarely considered in the legal and ethical literature on competency: The consent process must conclude with the patient's expressing his or her choice of medical treatment.

These points cover capability to participate in the doctor-patient game, as that game is played within our society. Should any further requirement be added on behalf of authorization? Or, since our society values freedom and autonomy so highly, should anyone capable of consenting to treatment be authorized to do so? I argued that another factor is required, which I termed "recognizable reasons." Competency to consent would then require that a patient understand the choice that needs to be made, make a choice, and be capable of providing reasons for having made that choice that others may recognize as relevant, without necessarily agreeing with them.

As a practical matter, the "recognizable reasons" addendum would find that a patient is incompetent to consent if she is incapable of providing any reason for her choice or if the reason provided bears no relation to the choice made, that is, is a non sequitur, or if her reason relies upon a provably false proposition, clung to despite all evidence to the contrary (i.e., a delusion).

Why should a "recognizable reasons" proviso be added to the elements that ensure capability to consent? Within society, each of our actions impinges upon the lives of others, to a greater or lesser degree, thus forcing others to reorder their own lives and choices. Freedom of action within society is tolerable to the extent that the actions of those around me are to some degree predictable, to the extent that I can in some manner understand the motivated conduct of others and adjust my own activities accordingly. Within a society that values the free action of autonomous persons, a recognizable reasons proviso is needed to preserve freedom consistent with some degree of social order, because, by restricting free action to those persons who act in relatively predictable ways, more intrusive means of inducing predictability are rendered unnecessary.

A "recognizable reasons" proviso is particularly appropriate to a society of strangers, to the legal ordering of persons who encounter one another with no prior knowledge of the other. You meet a person for the first time who acts oddly. Is that person wicked, or eccentric, or mad? You have no baseline of previous behavior against which to compare the deeds of the person. You know nothing of the culture and values of this person, other than that they may be quite different from your own. You are restricted to trying to judge whether the person's behavior makes sense, hangs together, upon the other's own premises, whatever they may be. Without judging the wisdom of the other, you attempt to discern whether the other is acting in a way that can be rationally reconstructed.

A Midrash on the Social Representation of Madness

Consider the other side of the coin: Suppose you were meeting a stranger and you needed to prove to him that you are mad? How would you behave? Beyond simulating some classic symptoms of mental illness, you would affect an air of being—literally—beyond reason, of acting in ways that would strike the other as not merely strange (for strangeness is expected of the stranger), but truly incoherent. The Bible describes this as the problem faced, and the solution adopted, by David in his search for asylum in the Philistine city of Gat, at the time David was fleeing from King Saul:

> David arose and fled that day from before Saul; he arrived at Achish, king of Gat.
>
> The servants of Gat said to him, Is this not David, king of the land; is it not of him that they recite in dance, saying, Saul struck in his thousands, and David in his tens of thousands?
>
> David placed these words within his heart; he was greatly afraid of Achish, king of Gat.
>
> He feigned madness [va'y'shano et ta'amo] in their eyes, he raved in their hands; he scribbled on the doors of the gate, and dripped spittle upon his beard.
>
> Achish said to his servants; Behold, see, a man deranged, why do you bring him to me?
>
> Am I short of the insane, that you have brought this one to be deranged before me; shall this one come to my house?[69]

The biblical description is terse; a rabbinic commentary fills out background and details, and supplies a moral to the story:

> [Introducing this story, the Midrash writes,] Of this Scripture is said,[70] "Everything was made lovely in its own time": All that the Holy One Blessed Be He made in his world is lovely. He [David] had said before the Holy One: Master of the World: Everything you made in your world is lovely, and wisdom is loveliest of all—except for madness. What pleasure is there for a madman? A man walks in the market, and tears his garments, and children make fun of him and run after him, and the people make fun of him: Is this lovely before you?
>
> The Holy One said to David: David! Are you criticizing madness? By your life, you will have need of it, you will be in sorrow and you will pray for it until I shall give you of it. . . .
>
> [Returning to our story, v. 13:], At that time David was frightened, and began praying and saying, Master of the

world, respond to me at this time. The Holy One said to him, David, what are you requesting? He said: Give to me some of that of which we had spoken. He said: Did I not tell you that you would ask for madness?

He made himself like a madman, writing on the doors: Achish, king of Gat, owes me a million, and his wife five hundred thousand.

The daughter of Achish was a madwoman, and was shouting and behaving insanely from within, and David shouting and acting insanely from without. Achish said to them: Did you think that I have a dearth of mad people, as it says, Am I short of the insane? At that moment David rejoiced, as his madness left him from his rejoicing; of this it is written,[71] "I shall bless G-d on every occasion."[72]

With this Midrashic interpolation, the biblical scene acquires cinematic vividness. David seeks asylum incognito, but is recognized and brought before the king. His situation is not good: The king, Achish, may return him to Saul, who will put him to death. Alternatively, Achish may put David to death himself: In the portion of the Midrash omitted here, the servants of Achish urge this course of action upon him as punishment for David's having slain Achish's brother, Goliath. David, ever resourceful, responds by feigning madness—in effect, by pleading insanity. David is to learn that madness, too, is needed in its proper time: as a basis for negating responsibility.

How does he feign madness? As the Bible relates, he rants, and raves, and scrawls, and drools—revolting, unselfconscious action. The Midrash, as is its wont, fills in the gap, answering the unasked question: But what did he scribble? David's behavior in the Midrash's recension will be familiar to anyone today with experience with mental illness as the characteristic grandiosity of paranoia: "Achish, king of Gat, owes me a million, and his wife five hundred thousand."

Most revealing, however, is the phrase the Bible uses that was translated as "feigning madness," viz., *vay'shano et ta'amo*. This means, literally, he changed or lost his *ta'am;* and *ta'am* in turn, which refers generally to reason, has a specific meaning when spoken by David:

rationality in action, deeds that are well-ordered to express a value or achieve a goal. For example: Later in the biblical tale, David proposes to kill the treacherous Naval and all of his men. He is dissuaded by reasons offered by Avigayil, to whom David then says, "And blessed is your *ta'am* and blessed are you."[73]

The effective presentation of mental illness between strangers requires overt, floridly psychotic behavior. And, in a culture of strangers with limited or no responsibility toward the other, the license to freely play the social role that is competency may not be denied on lesser grounds. There, the bare capability to exercise social roles is simply the capability to effectively exercise rights, and any added requirement on behalf of authorization will be minimal (as in the recognizable reasons addendum), itself justified because of its furtherance of the personal scope of freedom. Within a social regimen of neighbors, which assigns central value to duty, it is otherwise. The important social roles to be filled are defined by duty, and, as we all learn in struggling to fulfill obligations, capability to perform a duty may be far more onerous than capability to exercise a right.

Conclusion: The General Theory of Competency in Society Today and Tomorrow

Yet in our socikey, as in any society, the elements of competency must respond to changes in the social context. We should acknowledge that any current understanding is temporary and may need to be reexamined and revised in light of changes, both factual and valuational. If we think of a grant of competency as a limited license to freely act in an important social role, we must be particularly alert to changes in the nature and implications of those social roles themselves.

As the nature and implications of medical treatment are particularly prone to change, we should consider whether its associated competence needs to be reexamined. In 1850, understanding the nature and consequences of a proposed treatment and its alternatives did not require much effort on the part of a patient. Treatments were simple; what was known of their consequences, little; alternatives, few. Informed consent today—and a patient's capability to utilize the doctrine of informed consent—has become hard because of a confluence of trends: an exploding pharmacopoeia and the proliferation of alternatives such as surgery or preventive care, ever more finely grained knowledge about the pathways of healing and of side effects associated with interventions; increased alertness to long-term consequences of treatment; a growing range of conditions that are amenable to effective intervention, all going hand in hand with a lowered public threshold of tolerance for disease and disability.

Reproductive technology exemplifies these points well. Infertility was transformed from a personal tragedy into a disease once our understanding of its causes and ability to reverse them grew. Early, simple interventions by large doses of fertility drugs were seen in retrospect to be too clumsy and risky. Over time, reproductive technology has offered an ever-increasing number of alternative interventions. But this progress has fed rather than satisfied a public appetite for the total control and timing of reproduction.

These trends have accelerated rather than peaked. It is undoubtedly a gross underestimate to predict that the complexity of medical choices in 2150 will be as far beyond those of today as today's are of those of 1850.

All this speaks only to the bare capability to comprehend and meaningfully choose among medical options. We should consider as well whether authorization needs to be reexamined in a society of ever-growing interdependency, for example, in a context of rising health care costs whose payment is made or defrayed by third parties, particularly government. Crudely put, if health care choices impact financially upon society, license to freely choose treatments arguably should be restricted by society to those who can do this skillfully and with prudent foresight—to those who substantially exceed in skill the bare capability to play the "patient game."

I end this chapter by noting that our reaction to these changes and reexamination of competency in their light will call for empathy and imagination as well as analytic clarity. Competency to hold a job has changed in ways very similar to competency to consent to treatment. The intensity and length of education, as well as degree of literacy, numeracy, and technological ability required for jobs today—in agriculture, manufacturing, and office work, as well as in the professions—far exceed those required by their counterparts 150 years past, and again, the trends show no sign of diminishing. Society has reacted, unimaginatively, by simply raising the threshold of occupational competence, a choice that has resulted in massive and growing job dislocations and unemployment. The cost of this social choice of occupational competency has been high, and arguably would be higher yet in association with a "job" even more intimately personal and necessary—the choice of medical treatment.

It may be argued that although some formal aspects of defining competency are universal (for example, the need to define competency's minimal conditions), Judaism has little to teach us about the moral dilemmas and social problems associated with substantive competency. The Jewish view, embedded within a framework of duties and obligations (similar to the early common law's emphasis upon status), has no relevance to the contemporary approach, within which individual autonomy is the preeminent value, so that competent choice trumps competing interests.[74] The last points made argue to the contrary. As was true of the Jewish approach, any theory of competency needs to be constructed in awareness of social realities as well as values. In a sense, this is even more true the more a society values maximizing autonomy, for competency serves then as a license for the *free* exercise of power on the part of citizens. As technology and communications advance, enhancing the power of individuals and extending their reach, society needs to reconsider the effects of allowing unfettered choice. One major arena within which that reconsideration must take place, I believe, is in the very definition and scope of competency itself.

Endnotes

1. Loren H. Roth, Alan Meisel, and Charles W. Lidz, "Tests of Competency to Consent to Treatment," *American Journal of Psychiatry* 134 (1977): 279–284.

2. See Allen E. Buchanan and Dan W. Brock, *Deciding for Others* (New York: Cambridge University Press, 1989).*

3. James Drane, "The Many Faces of Competency," *Hastings Center Report* 15, no. 2 (1985): 17–21.*

4. Compare with Buchanan and Brock (1989): 23–24.

5. TB *Gitin*, 67b.

6. TB *Gitin*, 70b.

7. It has been authoritatively codified as law: cf. *Tur, Even Ha'ezer,* 121.

8. I am grateful to my friend and colleague, Prof. Stan Shapiro, for this analogy.

9. Thanks again to Prof. Stan Shapiro.

10. Andrew Kertesz, 1982; distributed by the Psychological Corporation.

11. I am grateful to Gail Poole for suggesting this point.*

12. An interesting side issue I will not pursue here concerns the nature of this knowledge and its manner of demonstration.*

13. See Richard J. Bonnie, "Medical Ethics and the Death Penalty," *Hastings Center Report* 20, no. 3 (1990): 12–18.*

14. See Milton D. Green, "Public Policies Underlying the Law of Mental Incompetency," *Michigan Law Review* 38 (1940): 1189–1221, at 1204.*

15. See Green (1940); see also Green's "Judicial Tests of Mental Incompetency," *Missouri Law Review* 6 (1941): 141–165, at 154–155.*

16. See Green (1940): 1203, 1209.*

17. James F. Drane, "Competency to Give an Informed Consent: A Model for Making Clinical Assessments," *Journal of the American Medical Association* 252 (1984): 925–927.

18. See Green (1940, 1941); see also his "Fraud, Undue Influence and Mental Incompetency—A Study in Related Concepts," *Columbia Law Review* 43 (1943): 176–205; and "Proof of Mental Incompetency and the Unexpressed Major Premise," *Yale Law Journal* 53 (1943): 271–311.

19. See P. Deschamps, K. C. Glass, B. M. Knoppers, and B. Morneault, *Health Care Liability in Canada* (Quebec Research Centre of Private and Comparative Law, 1989).

20. TB *Gitin* 59a.

21. Article 172 of the Quebec Civil Code.

22. Article 174; my thanks to Maître Lazar Sarna for providing this reference.

23. Rambam, *Mishne Tora, Sefer Kinyan, Hilkhot M'khira,* 29.6–8.

24. See Responsa Rivash 20, and the talmudic source, TB *Bava Batra* 155.*

25. Compare with Mishna, TB *Y'vamot* 112b.*

26. TY *Y'vamot* 14b, ch. 14, Law 1.

27. Deut. 24.3.

28. TB *Y'vamot* 113b.

29. See *Tosfot,* Rabbenu Asher, and *Korban N'tanel* on the Babylonian passage; Rambam, *Mishne Tora, Hilkhot Gerushin,* ch. 10.23; Responsa *Achi'ezer,* part 3, section 17; Responsa *Sridei Esh,* part 3, section 1, s.v. *v'achshav;* Responsa Maharshal 65; and Responsa *Yeshu'ot Malko,* excerpts from Responsa, section 3.*

30. Responsa *Meishiv Davar,* part 4, section 45.

31. Gaius, D. 24.21.1, cited in Boaz Cohen, *Jewish and Roman Law,* vol. 1 (New York: Jewish Theological Seminary, 1966): 387.

32. Colin M. Turnbull, *The Mountain People* (New York: Simon & Schuster, 1972).*

33. Compare with *Tur Even Ha'ezer* 119.

34. This interpretation is discussed but rejected in *Tosfot Y'vamot* 113b, s.v. *yatzta;* something similar to it was adopted by Responsa Maharshal 65 and Responsa *Meishiv Davar,* part 4, section 45.

35. Yigael Yadin, *Bar-Kokhba* (New York: Random House, 1971): 222, 237, 239.

36. Contrast with the view expressed in the Jerusalem Talmud by R Nechemia bar Mar Ukvan b'rei d'R Yosi.*

37. See TB *Gitin* 38b; see also Rambam, above; Responsa *Achi'ezer,* part 3, section 17.*

38. See Responsa Maharshal 65.*

39. Green (1940): 1216, note 98. See also Green (1943): 183.*

40. TB *Chagiga* 2a.

41. TB *Chagiga* 3b–4a.

42. TY *T'rumot* 1.1, p. 40b.

43. R Abraham Dor Levin, "The Illnesses of a *Shote* and of *Shtut* in Jewish Law," in *Halakha Urfu'a,* vol. 4, ed. Rav Moshe Hershler (Chicago and Jerusalem: Regensburg Institute, 1985): 263–269.

44. See, e.g., *Otzar Haposkim,* end of part 2, p. 22.

45. See discussion in Moshe Halevi Spero, *Handbook of Psychotherapy and Jewish Ethics* (Jerusalem: Feldheim, 1986): 74, note 53, and his Appen-

dix II: "Cognitive/Emotional Presentations and *Halakha:* A Typological Index in re Mental Incompetence."

46. See Marcus Jastrow, *A Dictionary of the Targumin* (reprinted in Israel by Hillel Press, no date), s.v. *hamarah.*

47. This interpretation is strengthened by noting the occurrence in rabbinic literature of the less-frequent syndromes, *hamarah halvanah* and *hamarah ha'adumah,* the white and red *hamarah,* respectively.*

48. See Levin, note 43 *supra.**

49. Revised Standard Version Luke 8.27; compare also Mark 5.5 on this tale.

50. See Julius Preuss, *Biblical and Talmudic Medicine,* trans. Fred Rosner (New York: Hebrew Publishing Company, 1978): 317.

51. Rambam, *Hilkhot Eidut,* 9.9.

52. See *Hilkhot Yesodei Hatorah* 5.11; see also *Hilkhot Issurei Bi'a* 6.4; for other examples, see *Hilkhot Eiruvin* 3.15; *Hilkhot Shofar veSukka veLulav* 5.14.*

53. Compare with *Hilkhot Akum.**

54. *Per contra,* see Isadore Twersky, *Introduction to the Code of Maimonides* (New Haven, CT: Yale University Press, 1980).*

55. TY *T'rumot* 1.1.

56. For confirmation, see Responsa *Ein Yitzchak* 2, *Even Ha'ezer,* section 9, s.v. *V'od.**

57. This obscure illness was identified by Rashi.*

58. An acute confusional state in reaction to alcohol.

59. Compare, for example, TB *Shabbat* 88a.*

60. Responsa *Chatam Sofer* 4, *Even Ha'ezer* 2, section 2.

61. *Derekh Eretz Zuta,* the beginning of chapter 9.

62. TB *Yoma,* 20b–21a.

63. TB *Nida* 17a.

64. Eisenstein, *Otzar Hamidrashim* 162, s.v. *Gimel hiti'akh.*

65. Rambam's language was a cause of consternation to his commentators, the *Nos'ei Kelim,* who thought the reason he provided should have been a lack of understanding on the part of the *shote,* rather than an absence of obligation.*

66. TB *Chagiga* 2a.

67. See Benjamin Freedman, "Competence, Marginal and Otherwise: Concepts and Ethics," *International Journal of Law and Psychiatry* 4 (1981): 53–72. Also see the final report of the province of Ontario's Clark Committee on law reform and the use of electroconvulsive therapy.

68. See Miriam Siegler and Humphrey Osmond, *Models of Madness, Models of Medicine* (New York: Macmillan, 1974).

69. I Sam. 21.11–16.

70. Eccl. 3.11.

71. Ps. 34.2.

72. *Yalkut Shim'oni* on I Sam. 21, comment 131.

73. I Sam. 25.33.*

74. I am indebted to Prof. Richard Bonnie for presenting this counter-argument.

RISK

principles of judgment in health care decisions

Introduction

In the previous chapters I have tried to explain how a regime of duty such as Judaism must retain, in some form, the doctrine of informed consent. As a reasonable, responsible caretaker of her own body, held in trust for G-d, a person is allowed and even required to investigate her medical options and to arrive at an informed and appropriate treatment decision. For those *shotim,* persons who are legally incompetent precisely because (as we have seen) they are unable to discharge the duty to care for the self, proxy decision makers such as family members are similarly charged.

This chapter deals with the question: How is the appropriateness of a treatment decision determined? Is it possible, in general, to define a set of characteristics that will make a particular decision the right decision for a patient? We have already considered in the context of consent one approach to this question, that the patient is required to conform in all cases and in all respects to the physician's recommendation. As stated by R Yechiel Mechal Tukatchinski:

> Once the physician has done his part, and placed before him [the patient] the laws of medicine, and the behavior and nutrition that he requires—the patient is *duty-bound* [*chayav;* emphasis in original] to obey the doctor's orders, no less and no more than the laws of the *Shulchan Arukh* [Code of Jewish Law] concerning the prohibited and the permitted, as a *mitzva* of the Torah: "You shall take great care of your souls."[1]

This approach, grounded in the view that in general a medical recommendation expresses a clear and unique treatment approach that is unambiguously in the patient's interest, was rejected. More typically, a health care decision is made under conditions of uncertainty, requires a weighing of costs and risks as well as prospective benefits, and consequently involves a range of responsible choice. But the moral question still remains: When making health care decisions, what risks and harms are a reasonable caretaker permitted to undergo, under what circumstances, and to what ends?

Jewish tradition affords a variety of principles to deal with this question, which will be the subject of this chapter. As before, while the material to be presented is largely drawn from Jewish sources, I believe it has more than parochial interest. Any religious or moral tradition that maintains that persons have self-regarding obligations, or, as some traditions put it, must express stewardship in their decisions, faces together with normative Judaism the question of how to discharge these duties in the health care realm. My discussion will be limited to this personal ethical issue and is not primarily concerned with the question of when, if ever, a patient may be *compelled* to act responsibly or to undergo treatment that he or she was duty bound to accept. Also, because this study is restricted to the self-regarding obligations of the reasonable caretaker, I will not deal with the important topic of other-regarding obligations and self-sacrifice. Finally, as has been true throughout this book on the elements of a Jewish bioethic, I will not explore such complicated questions as arise, for example, when one principle conflicts with another.

Why Is Life-Prolonging Treatment Refused? Two Cases

The following consultation notes concern two cases similar to those dealt with in the sources I will present later. The first case involves a patient's refusal of recommended treatment, the second, refusal on behalf of a patient by a proxy. Both cases present fairly dramatic, life-and-death decisions, as does much of the Jewish literature itself. And both raise the basic question of responsible stewardship: Under what circumstances and for what reasons may a person responsibly refuse a medical recommendation?

ETHICS CONSULTATION: A PATIENT'S INSTRUCTIONS
FOR NO-CODE AND A PHYSICIAN'S DENIAL

Mr. S is a seventy-eight-year-old man in the coronary care unit. He had just undergone a balloon angioplasty [a surgical procedure to open a blocked or narrowed artery of the heart]. He was described to me on the phone as fully alert and competent. Mr. S had instructed his doctor and others in the unit that in the event of an arrest or sudden worsening of his condition, he does not wish to be resuscitated or intubated. Upon hearing of these instructions, Dr. T, the surgeon who had performed the angioplasty, insisted that the patient is to be "full code" for at least the next twenty-four hours. The purpose of the consultation, requested by Dr. V, the responsible cardiologist on the unit, was to clarify the patient's code status in that light.

I came and spoke with Mr. S, together with Dr. V, as noted above. He is a pleasant, intelligent, caring, sensible, and sensitive man, concerned that his desires not inconvenience the staff. (At one point, in speaking of his wish not to be resuscitated, he qualified this by saying something like "Unless you really feel you have to because of your job.") He is determined that he not be a burden upon his family and that if his condition should worsen such that he will not recover independent function, he be allowed to die.

Mr. S was completely competent and appropriate in his manner of speech when I met him. Follow-up of Dr. T's surgical patients is done not by him but by the coronary care unit's staff, so I did not have the chance to speak with Dr. T. I cannot therefore comment upon his express refusal to abide by the patient's wishes. It is possible that he felt that since there was a heightened chance of reversible arrhythmia secondary to the angioplasty, it is inconsistent for a patient to agree to undergo the procedure and then to prospectively refuse a needed correction of this potential side effect. This is a reasonable stance for Dr. T to hold, and it is his right to try to convince the patient of its wisdom. There is, though, no question in my mind that legally and ethically the patient is entitled to have his wishes respected.

Discussion with Mr. S was fairly brief. He explained the intention underlying his decision and reiterated his wishes. I probed his desires somewhat, trying to ascertain whether there are procedures covered under his refusal that he might not necessarily wish to exclude. It appeared that his desires were predicated less upon aversion to resuscitative measures themselves than to a desire to not be treated if he will not be functional. After clarification, he agreed to a single effort at cardioversion should that become necessary, on the chance that his heartbeat might be easily recovered, but did not wish to go any further.

Patients may refuse treatment for any number of reasons: for example, because they don't think they are so ill as to need treatment, or because they fear the side effects of treatment, or because they simply don't believe treatment will work. I had guessed that Mr. S's refusal was of the second sort. Although families who insist that "everything must be done" for their relative do not realize this, cardiopulmonary resuscitation (CPR) is far from the clean, painless, bloodless medical intervention that television dramas often make it appear. My guess, that Mr. S wanted to be spared the staged violence that CPR in fact requires, was wrong. His fear was a peculiarly modern one. He was afraid that resuscitation would in fact be successful—but not successful enough. He refused CPR because he thought it would restore him to a crippled, helpless, bedridden life. Setting aside the accuracy of this judgment (I thought his prospects in the event of an arrest were neither as gloomy as he thought nor as rosy as Dr. T may believe), one question Mr. S's decision poses is: Is it responsible for a patient to choose to forgo the possibility of benefit for fear of a bad result? The following, rather puzzling case plays a variation on the same question.

Ethics Consultation: Father and Sons

A ninety-eight-year-old man—described by Dr. N, a senior neurologist, as "one of our patients in late adolescence"—was suffering from a bilateral subdural hematoma ["bruise," a collection of blood and other fluids between the brain and skull, on both sides of the head] resulting from a fall he had experienced in the previous winter. He required a reduction by burr-holes [a surgical procedure to drain the hematoma]. His two sons, one of whom lives in Florida and the other of whom is still in Montreal (both of whom appear to be in their seventies), were refusing to consent to this relatively simple operation.

Until the fall, the elder Mr. M. was an active, alert man: mobile, taking walks every day, dabbling in the stock market. His deteriorating condition was not recognized, save in retrospect, as resulting from a significant event. (He had in fact been investigated immediately following the fall at another city hospital that had failed to rule out subdural hematoma via CT scan.) Over the following months he lost mobility and alertness and was diagnosed as succumbing to dementia. At the present time, he was receiving artificial support in the hospital and was no longer communicative at all.

In sessions Mr. M's son held with Dr. N, with Dr. N and myself, and finally with me alone—amounting to several hours of meeting time in all—the medical situation was outlined for them. It was possible—quite likely—that he would die regardless of the procedure, or even as a result of the procedure; and possible that he would survive in an impaired state. Most relevantly, Dr. N thought it was entirely possible that he could recover to baseline, that is, to the level of functioning the patient had enjoyed prior to becoming ill. Dr. N's "guesstimate" of the relative odds of these outcomes was given, rather loosely, as "low" in the case of death during the procedure ("maybe 10%"), and evenly divided as between impaired and fully functional survival.

Given that, the refusal by the sons was puzzling. They appeared to me to be in every way intelligent men who loved their father and wanted to defend his best interests. Yet, I could get no clear reason for their refusal. I was told that he is old, that he has suffered enough, that he wouldn't want this, etc., but each reason offered was unstable (i.e., abandoned when we focused our discussion on it). Also, the sons did not even attempt to consider, and respond to, the reasons why Dr. N felt to the contrary.

For Dr. N, a decision not to operate in this case would be nothing less than age discrimination: A man thirty years younger but with the identical diagnosis and prognosis would be operated upon without any question, and a refusal by next of kin would be overridden. I was inclined to side with Dr. N on this.

As near as I could make out, there were two important factors operating to sustain their refusal. First, over a period of months they had accustomed themselves to the idea that he was in irreversibly failing health due to dementia, and they found it difficult or impossible to re-gear their thinking or decision making. Second, they wanted the decision to be taken out of their hands, and found that by refusing to consent to the surgery they could escape responsibility.

Late in a private discussion with them, when I thought they were about to change their minds (or at any rate were wavering), one asked me what would happen if they still refused. I said that in that case I would talk to the hospital's Director of Professional Services (DPS), and tell him that he ought to consider contacting the office of the public guardian for authority to perform the procedure; and that, in all likelihood, he would so act and the office would approve the operation. After telling them that, they said, "Well, I guess that's what you'll have to do then." They were not at all angry at me for thwarting their desires, and in fact were both pleasant and grateful to me for taking so much time with them on this.

Given this last point, I was left uncertain as to what I would do in the next such case. In particular, knowing that talking about what we would do may give family members an out, should they be left off the hook in this way? I think probably they should—they should be left free to escape responsibility in whatever fashion they find most natural or least threatening— but I am still quite unsure.

This case, which took place some time ago, remains vivid in my mind for several reasons: Coming early in my work at that institution, it was the first time that I was involved in an attempt to override the wishes of a patient's next of kin (something that as a legal matter was much simpler then than it is now). The patient was the oldest patient on which I had consulted at that time, and the patient's children were the oldest "patient's children" with which I had dealt. Coming to meet them for the first time, confronted by two gentlemen in their seventies—with one dressed in "full Florida," from white shoes to white belt to white golf cap—I thought I had come to the wrong room: All of the patient's children with whom I dealt previously were middle-aged.

And I remember it for its outcome. I did meet with the hospital's DPS, who agreed with my assessment and immediately sought legal authority for the procedure. (He knew better than I that Dr. N is by no means "quick on the trigger," and was impressed that a physician who is generally very conservative in ordering procedures was adamant that this operation be done.) The scheduled burr-hole reduction was delayed by two days. In the interim, Mr. M experienced an apparently unconnected coronary event, which proved irreversible, and died. In the end, his children were right to refuse, although perhaps for the wrong reasons.

In the following sections, I will explore some lines of reasoning that have been developed in Jewish sources to clarify decisions about health care that involve risk. Traditionally, normative Judaism has been exceedingly risk-averse, preferring in every case to err, if error it will be, on the side of life:

> One who had a structure fall upon him [on the Sabbath], and it is uncertain whether he is there or not, whether he is dead or alive, whether he is Cuthite or Jew, the heap is cleared off of him [despite the Sabbath violation this involves]: If they found him living they continue clearing, if he is dead they leave him [until after the Sabbath].[2]

> In matters of preserving life, we do not follow majorities [i.e., rely upon probabilities].[3]

Yet even this tradition has recognized the necessity for allowing a degree of personal judgment, of choice—even of style—to operate. I will be emphasizing the scope for choice that some sources of normative Judaism tolerate, as a corrective to the received view expressed here by R Tukatchinski, among many others. Nevertheless, it is clear that in a regime of duty such as Judaism, such choices are subject to strict moral constraint. From the Jewish point of view, as our bodies are not our own property, our choices need to be validated by more than simple personal preference. In general, these sources follow the principle that risks must be counterbalanced by proportional gains, so that even the gravest risks are allowable under extreme conditions.

Allowable Risks I:
Risking Life to Lengthen Life

The first such principle we will examine arises out of the most extreme circumstances: A person who is to die shortly may risk immediate death on behalf of the prospect of lengthened life. One of the earliest rabbinic discussions of this issue is found in Responsa *Sh'vut Ya'akov*, written by R Ya'akov Reisher (ca. 1670–1733):

> [Question:] From an expert physician regarding a person who has fallen ill, and is close to dying from his sickness. All of the physicians estimate that he will certainly die within one or two days. However, they judge that there is one further treatment that could possibly heal his illness. It is also possible that, to the contrary, if he takes this treatment and it is unsuccessful, he may, G-d forbid, die immediately, within one or two hours. Is it permitted to perform this treatment; or, do we concern ourselves over fleeting life *[chayei sha'a]*, and it is preferable to refrain from acting?
>
> Response: Since this law is truly one of life and death, one needs to be very cautious in its regard, considering the Talmud and rabbinic decisions with seven inquiries and investigations. For, anyone who causes the loss of the life of any Jew etc. [is considered as though he had destroyed an entire world], and so too the opposite: Anyone who preserves the life of another is considered as though he had preserved an entire world. And at first glance, it appeared as though refraining from acting is preferable, for we do concern ourselves over fleeting life, and even one who is already moribund *[goses]*.
>
> . . . When I descended into the analysis, it appeared acceptable. . . . If it is possible that by means of the treatment

that he [the doctor] provides to him, he will be completely cured of his sickness, then we certainly do not concern ourselves over fleeting life. There is a clear proof of this found in a talmudic discussion. . . .

. . . In this matter, since he would certainly die, we cast aside the certainty and grasp at a possibility, that he may be healed. But in any event, the doctor should not do this as an easy matter. He must act with great deliberation, and should clarify whether the expert physicians of the city, by a majority opinion—i.e., by a great majority, namely, a two-to-one margin—[support this treatment approach or not] since we must be concerned that some people act lightly. Therefore, he should act according to the majority view of the physicians, and the approval of the Sage of the city.[4]

Patient Choice of Treatment: Setting the *Halakhic* Stage

The idea of "being concerned" (or "worried," "fearful," "troubled": *chay'y'shinan*) over some issue is central to a Jewish approach, or indeed to any ethical analysis of a case of conscience. When we ask if we "are concerned" about fleeting life, for example, we ask whether this is a factor that must be taken into account in our decision making. Ethics, being practical philosophy—that is, concerned with our practice and actions rather than simply beliefs—"takes account" of factors when they are recognized as having the potential to convince us to act in one way rather than another. Certainly, not every aspect and consequence of every action can be admitted to the realm of ethical deliberation, or ethical analysis would be a prescription for paralysis. Different ethical theories will highlight certain of these for attention, "concern": for example, the pain an action will cause, or whether an action is fair or just.

Here, by asking whether we "are concerned" over fleeting life, the author is asking whether the danger that this treatment poses, that a patient's death will be advanced by one or two days, should convince us that such a treatment is prohibited. Arguing in favor of this view is the innate conservatism of duty. By refraining from an action, nature is allowed to take its course, and it is nature, his illness, that is killing this patient. Fleeting life, of a day or two's duration, is still of value in Jewish law. "A single [law applies] to one who murders a healthy person or murders an ill person who is languishing to death, and even one who murdered one who was moribund *[goses]:* He is killed for this [act]."[5] The permissions noted earlier to violate the Sabbath on behalf of a person buried under rubble who may or may not be alive hold equally on behalf of a person who retains only fleeting life. This "concern" that we express on behalf of fleeting life could therefore be expressed by invoking the principle that "it is preferable to refrain from acting," or literally rendered, "sit and do not act" *[shev v'al ta'ase]*.

Our author chose another way. He sets the stage for his decision by positing this case as a dilemma, a situation in which two choices are open, each of which is from one moral point of view preferable and, from another point of view, inferior, even sinful. He invokes the well-known rabbinic homily that states that the reason G-d founded the human race by forming a single being, Adam, was to teach that anyone who kills a single person is considered as one who has destroyed an entire world, and, contrariwise, that one who saves another is considered as though he or she had saved a complete world. The precedents must be very closely investigated, he writes, for there is as much praise associated with saving another as there is blame connected with killing the other. In this situation of risk, these two principles pull in opposing directions: The patient cannot be saved without chancing his destruction. Significantly, he rules that in this type of case the duty to save life overrides the duty to refrain from endangering life.

A Crucial Recognition: There Is No Way to "Play It Safe"

The passive advice "sit and do not act" is appropriate to circumstances in which, by refraining from action, you avoid the chance of violating the law (while at the same time you lose the chance of performing some meritorious act). The acceptable is embraced, and the better is eschewed for fear of doing evil. Do not, however, be deceived. To "sit" is, after all, to do *something*. "Sit and do not act" is inappropriate advice when by the very act of "sitting" you chance the violation of one duty, the duty to rescue the life of another, at the very same time as you obviate the chance that another duty may be infringed.

The crux of the decision of *Sh'vut Ya'akov*, to permit the dangerous medical intervention, follows from his recognition that the case posed represents a clash of duties. There is no way to "play it safe" from the ethical point of view here, just as there is no way to "err on the side of life"; for ethics, and life, may be mobilized to support either one of two opposed courses of action. This same step is taken by R Eli'ezer Waldenberg, invoking the reasoning of a previous authority. Speaking of the permissibility of another form of dangerous surgery (in fact, psychosurgery), he writes,

I noticed in the volume *Sefer Hachayim* of R Sh Kluger,[6] that within his response he provides a further novel reason to permit this [a dangerous operation], provided the sick person himself consents to accept upon himself the responsibility to endanger himself. This is because: While it is true that a person does not have the authority to kill himself, and if he kills himself he is [guilty of] intentionally committing suicide, nevertheless it appears that intentional suicide itself is [regulated by] nothing more than a positive commandment, learned by the rabbis from the verse, "yet your blood of your souls I shall seek." If so, this positive commandment itself is suppressed *[nidche]* on behalf of the rescue of a soul *[piku'ach nefesh]*. Just as the Sabbath is suppressed on account of rescue, and even on the strength of a possibility of rescue, so too here this positive commandment of "yet your blood from your souls" is suppressed on account of rescue, and even of a doubtful rescue,—for this positive commandment [to guard your own life] is no more stringent than the Sabbath.[7]

Patient Choice: Talmudic Roots

R Ya'akov Reisher had found precedent for his ruling in the following talmudic discussion:

[Various persons testify that] R Yochanan said: If there is a chance he [a sick person] may live, and a chance he may die, he may not be treated by them [idol-worshipers who treat the sick]. [Rashi explains: For an idolater will certainly murder him, and it is preferable that he remain with the possibility that he will live.] If he will certainly die, he may be treated by them. [Rashi: In a case in which we know that if not treated he will certainly die, and there is no Jew present to treat him, he is treated by them. For, what is the idolater to do to him? Without this he will die, and perhaps the idolater will heal him.]

—"If he will die?" But there yet remains fleeting life [*chayei shá'a*]!

——We do not concern ourselves with fleeting life.

And where do we learn that we do not concern ourselves with fleeting life? It is written,[8] "If we say we will go to the city, and famine is in the city, we will die there." Yet, there remained fleeting life! This proves nothing else than that we do not concern ourselves over fleeting life.[9]

Idol worship in talmudic times was viewed by the rabbis as being a "symptom" as much as a "disease." It marked off those persons who had chosen to reject minimal civilized norms of society. One who worshiped idols was presumptively a thief, an adulterer, and even a murderer as well.[10] In treating a patient, such a villain has even more scope for the expression of his antisocial impulses, for a doctor can clandestinely kill a patient without exciting suspicion, particularly if the patient is so ill that his life is endangered by his sickness.[11]

(A fascinating comparison emerges from the proceedings of the council of Avignon in 1337. In the early 1300s, ordinances began to appear restricting the right of Jewish physicians to attend to Christian patients. The reason initially given (in Provençal in 1306) was a concern that these doctors would not see to it that patients receive the last rites. Shortly thereafter (Valladodid, 1322; Salamanca, 1335) further reasons were advanced: Jewish doctors and apothecaries would kill

Christians under the guise of treatment. The Avignon council therefore stated,

> We establish and ordain that no Christian from our provinces, cities, and diocese of whatever status, condition, or dignity he may be, should approach and ask, or make us ask, any Jewish physician or surgeon for any medicine, medicament, or cure to be received from him. Neither should he dare to accept for himself, or through an intermediary person, any medicine, counsel, or cure coming from a Jew, or spontaneously sent by one, however excellent it may be, unless imminent danger to the patient exists and it is impossible to appeal conveniently to Christian doctors or surgeons.

An ensuing shortage of medical care led to repeal of this ordinance in 1341.)[12]

In modern terms, the Talmud is posing a case like one in which a person practicing medicine has been repeatedly charged with violent felonies, but has secured acquittal in each case on technical grounds. If no other were available, would you go to such a doctor? The Talmud's answer is, of course, it depends. You may not go to him if you have any other, safer option; you may, if you have nothing to lose. But, the Talmud objects, you do have something to lose: the brief life you currently enjoy. To this, the final response is: Fleeting life is no "concern" in this case, as is proven by biblical precedent.

Patient Choice: Biblical Roots

The verse fragment quoted, put in full, is as follows:

2 Kings 7
 3: And four men who were lepers were at the gates of the city; and each one said to his neighbor, Why do we sit here until we die?
 4: If we say we will go to the city, and the famine is in the city, then we will die there, and if we stay here we will die;

now, let us go and flee to the war camp of Aram, if they let us survive we will live, and if they kill us we will die.

The previous chapter had recounted the terrible famine in this city of Shomron, besieged by the army of Aram. In that chapter, a mother calls out to the king to save them and tells him how she has been approached by others to join a pact to share in the cannibalizing of their children; at the tale, the king tore his garments in grief and mourning.

These four leprous men of the city of Shomron were not "in" the city but "at its gates," in obedience, as commentators point out, to the Torah law requiring lepers to live outside of the city in isolation. These lepers faced, then, a threefold choice: They could stay at the gates of the city, as the Torah requires of lepers, and die of starvation; they could violate the Torah and enter the city, and die of starvation there; or they could go to the camp of the enemy. They chose to go to the enemy camp, risking the likelihood that a guard would simply run them through upon their approach, on behalf of the outside chance that the enemy soldiers would take mercy upon them and feed them.

Implications of the Precedents: Parameters of Patient Choice

This is the talmudic passage, with its associated biblical reference, relied upon by *Sh'vut Ya'akov* (and many subsequent authorities) in support of the proposition that a seriously ill patient may undergo a dangerous procedure. In later discussions, the lesson the Talmud taught is adapted in several different ways; we should therefore pause to consider what precisely this source states, and what issues are raised.

The time frame is uncertain, but seems very short. In the biblical tale, the lepers face death from starvation. Given the length and depth of the siege of the city, one may presume that the death they face will come within days, if not hours. The Talmud's lesson is not, however, specific on this point. The operative factor the Talmud states in presenting the law is not time but rather certainty: Only if one will certainly die may one approach this idolater for treatment; no time is specified.

In the talmudic discussion, however, as we have seen, some temporal dimension is implied, by the objection that in accepting treatment the patient risks his *chayei sha'a*. When the Talmud responds that we need not concern ourselves with *chayei sha'a*, it is possible, although not necessary, to infer the contrapositive, namely, that for something more than *chayei sha'a* we do indeed "concern ourselves." This term, which I have translated as "fleeting life," means literally "an hour's life." Its counterpart is *chayei 'olam*, which I will translate as "lasting life," although its literal meaning is "eternal life."[13]

In the responsum of *Sh'vut Ya'akov* we remain close to the biblical precedent, at any rate. The patient he discusses will live for twenty-four to forty-eight hours without treatment but will die in one to two hours if treatment is unsuccessful. Later commentators, however, have extended the period, while recognizing that this does violence to the literal signification of the term. R Moshe Feinstein, for example, who had prohibited the practice of heart transplantation in a 1968 responsum, stating of the perpetrators that "they are not concerned for his [the patient's] continued living, that is only an hour's life *[rak chayei sha'a]* or even some days' life,"[14] later elaborated the view that *chayei sha'a* encompasses anything up to twelve months' life.[15] And even twelve months does not represent an absolute limit; for, if a condition is not currently present but recurs intermittently and unpredictably and may become dangerous in a future recurrence, that too has been found to constitute grounds for the permitting of a dangerous operation.[16]

The action taken is a counsel of despair. In the biblical case of the lepers, while they seemed to face certain death from starvation were they to stay where they were, they faced very probable death upon approaching the enemy camp. (In fact, the story resumes with their discovery that the army was gone, the siege was broken, and grain once again is freely available.) The talmudic discussion, as understood by Rashi, posits as a near-certainty a murder attempt by the idolatrous physician: "For an idolater will certainly murder him," he writes. These are actions not taken out of reasonable expectation, but out of desperate hope, coupled with the certainty that nothing is lost by the gamble.

In *Sh'vut Ya'akov* there is no specification of likelihoods at all. We are not told whether the chances of success are considered low, high, or even, but we are told that the action is permitted. This became a source of contention for later writers. Is a dangerous operation permitted if its chances of successful cure are less than even? R Moshe Feinstein, for example, in one responsum, ruled that it is not.[17] Others allowed such an operation even if it held but a remote chance of success. This latter view seems closer to the lesson taught by the source material, and so was adopted by R Eli'ezer Waldenberg among others.[18]

The action seems permissible, at the patient's option, rather than compulsory. The language in the talmudic discussion is one of permission, rather than duty. We are told when the patient must not be healed by an idolater, but we are not told when he must acquiesce to such treatment. It seems to be the patient's option whether or not to approach the doctor. The issue is not dealt with at all in *Sh'vut Ya'akov,* but this is unsurprising: He was responding to a question raised by "an expert physician," who was apparently in the position to offer this treatment to a patient.

The biblical tale is interesting in this regard. By homiletic tradition, the four lepers were identified with Gechazi, an erstwhile servant of the prophet Elisha, and his sons. This Gechazi had imputed to him in rabbinic literature deep knowledge of the Torah. A description of his actions, therefore, might be taken as biblical warrant for the view that the choice he made is at least normatively acceptable, if not binding. At the same time, however, the Talmud states that Gechazi was so wicked that he forfeited his share in the World to Come![19]

Patient Medical Choice as an Expression of Patient Values

Noting the difficulty associated with taking Gechazi's actions as a normative model, R Moshe Feinstein reasons that the biblical passage was offered as an example, not as precedent; in the course of a remarkable discussion of the import of this example, R Feinstein sees this kind of choice (which he, however, restricts to cases in which the odds that the operation will cure or kill are even) as an expression of personal style:

> Therefore we have to say that R Yochanan says that the Torah law is in this instance dependent upon a person's judgment.

Since we see that for some persons a chance at prolonged life
[chayei gamur] is preferable to definite fleeting life, we say that
the Torah law permits [this choice; and the fact that Gechazi is
cited is just as an instance of this kind of judgment]. . . . It is
reasonable to say that for R Yochanan . . . there is in this case
ownership of a person over his own life to do that which is
good in his eyes for the sake of his life, for since we see that for
his good he is less concerned about fleeting life (so that he
would avoid being treated by an idolater because of the chance
that he may kill him right away), since there is in this hope for
prolonged life as people ordinarily experience as in the case of
their [the lepers] going to the war camp,—for in that case they
didn't worry that perhaps they would be killed and not live
even the days one can survive in spite of starvation. . . . These
two things [certain temporary life or doubtful prolonged life]
are both to his benefit [as opposed to someone who simply rejects temporary life]. . . . So we see in financial matters, there
are some who for a chance of a great profit buy merchandise
with the little money that they have even though if they do not
succeed they will lose the little they have; and there are some
who do not wish to buy [merchandise] with the little money
they have when there is a chance that they will lose their little:
Similarly it is possible that there is a division of opinion because of the nature of persons with respect to survival.[20]

I had reviewed this responsum shortly before the following case
consultation occurred; obviously, it had great resonance for me at that
time.

ETHICS CONSULTATION: NONVALIDATED TREATMENT IN STROKE

The patient is an eighty-year-old man who was brought back
from New York, where he had suffered a series of strokes in the
course of or following surgery. He has suffered great damage
from the strokes. He is bed- and chair-bound. He has sons who
have been given power of attorney, at least for financial matters,

who are much involved in his care at the hospital. His wife is at present overseas and so peripherally involved, though she remains in contact.

The question discussed concerned nonvalidated treatment (NVT). The patient, who in business and otherwise has been a frequent world traveler, has a long-standing relationship with a cardiologist from New York City. This cardiologist has attended his patient from time to time in Montreal in this current hospitalization. The cardiologist, who had, with Dr. A's knowledge, initiated—and subsequently, at Dr. A's direction, withdrawn—one form of NVT, involving heparin, has now proposed another NVT: urokinase at low doses, under the theory that it will dissolve the clots from the stroke. This treatment has no scientific basis, in the literature, animal studies, or otherwise and is lacking in a physiological rationale, since the damage from the strokes is now, months after the events, irreparable. Nevertheless, at the proposed doses, Dr. A feels the treatment is unlikely to cause the patient harm (keeping in mind the fact that any treatment, particularly under clinical rather than trial conditions, has the chance of producing unforeseen side effects).

I confirmed Dr. A's understanding that he is entirely within his rights as treating physician to refuse to allow this treatment; on the other hand, if he was comfortable with it, he could permit it, without going before the hospital's Research Ethics Board. Past experience in the hospital with patients and NVTs was briefly reviewed. Dr. A feels that he is broadly more favorable to offering NVTs to patients than many physicians, when—unlike in this case—he thinks it holds out hope. We spoke in terms of the level of a physician's comfort, but in these cases "comfort" is a surrogate term for the physician's own professional integrity and responsibility in treating a patient—no small thing.

One question I pursued had to do with the patient's history with this cardiologist. Had he previously, while competent, consented to NVTs under this physician, in full knowledge of its experimental nature? Had he done so, we might have a better understanding that that is what he would have wanted in these circumstances. Dr. A thought the patient probably had earlier received still more NVTs from this doctor. As a person and especially as a businessman, the patient had lived his life as a gambler—with, financially, great success—and Dr. A thought this could well have been the reason for an affinity between the patient and this particular cardiologist. He was much less sure that the cardiologist would have fully and frankly disclosed to his patient how little scientific support there was for such NVT. Like many other American physicians, the cardiologist is a bit of a salesman, emphasizing the positive and downplaying, if mentioning at all, the negative. I mentioned a responsum of Rabbi Moshe Feinstein, dealing with experimental and dangerous surgery, that made the same analogy as here, between risk-taking in business and in medical choices, and that reached the conclusion that a competent person's choice must be respected.

Dr. A plans to meet with the sons together with the cardiologist, so that a full airing of the issue might be made, and probably then to allow whatever the sons desire. I asked whether the patient himself might be communicative and competent enough to ratify a simple version of the decision, but after consideration, he felt that he is not. One final possibility that might be raised with the sons is that instead of a choice between conservative management and this particular NVT, they might consider instead enrolling the patient into an experimental protocol for stroke patients, here or elsewhere, that would have a stronger rationale and better chance for success than the NVT being proposed by the cardiologist.

When the Talmud had stated that we do not "concern ourselves" over fleeting life, *Tosfot* had noted—using some of the sources quoted earlier—that we do indeed weigh that factor heavily, for example, as a basis for permitting Sabbath violations. Their answer was that in every case we act to the patient's benefit. Excavating a person from rubble on the Sabbath is to his benefit, hence it is permitted; allowing a person who will otherwise die to risk his life for the chance of a cure is also to his benefit, hence it too is permitted. In other words, in these cases, a patient-centered risk-benefit analysis serves as the basis for determining whether an action is permissible, rather than some other automatic formula (such as "sit and do not act"). The very same consideration was straightforwardly applied by another contemporary scholar, R Shlomo Zalman Auerbach, asked by Prof. A. S. Abraham about the case of a fifty-year-old man suffering greatly from diabetes with serious complications including blindness and poor peripheral circulation. This has already caused gangrene and resulted in the amputation of one leg; the patient now has gangrene in the second leg.

> In consultation with the internists and surgeons together, it was concluded that this ill person will certainly die within a few days if his second leg were not to be amputated. However, he is likely as well to die in the course of the operation; and, of course, even if the operation should succeed and his fleeting life be prolonged, this treatment does not affect his underlying condition. The patient himself refused to undergo the operation because of fear of the operation itself, the pain and suffering it would cause, and basically because he did not wish to live as a blind double amputee. I then asked R Shlomo Zalman Auerbach the Torah's view of this case, and he ruled that the operation should not be performed against the patient's will (nor indeed should efforts be made to convince him to agree to the operation), since we are speaking of a major, risky procedure that will only add to the patient's suffering without any chance of gaining for him lasting life [chayei olam].[21]

What Is the Scope of Choice Open to the "Average, Reasonable Caretaker"?

What R Moshe Feinstein adds to this is the recognition that a judgment of what is to a patient's benefit is, to at least some extent, dependent upon that patient's own values and beliefs. Dr. A's patient, who is not presently competent to express his decision, has consistently lived the life of a gambler, indeed, of a high roller. These values are as well or better expressed in medical choices as in business judgments.

How do these sources stack up against the construct of "the average, reasonable caretaker"? They appear to me to give such a person the scope necessary to do the job properly. Rather than being restricted to the passive role of allowing nature to take its course ("sit and do nothing"), the patient is permitted to seek out alternatives and to actively experience a risk on behalf of a greater potential gain.[22]

In general, it seems to me, it would be impossible in theory to fault a caretaker who adheres to the results of a valid risk-benefit calculation, and who, weighing alternative treatments and their associated probabilities of length of life, chooses the one that promises the best outcome.[23] This statement assumes that other factors are equal. Two caveats must be introduced, arising from the possibilities that causing or allowing oneself to experience pain *[tza'ar]* and the same for "wounding" *[chavala]* are sources of wrong independent of danger. (These complications are discussed in the following sections.)

The difficulty lies in establishing that the risk-benefit calculation is indeed valid. Although written centuries ago, Ramban's classic exposition of medicine's risk and uncertainty, and the normative consequences that follow, remains valid:

> We should state it in this fashion: The doctor, even as the judge, is commanded to reach judgment. . . . The judge has nothing but that which his eyes see. . . . All this, provided that he is appropriately careful regarding these laws of life [Note: or, capital offenses—*dinei n'fashot*], and does not cause damage by negligence *[bip'shi'a]*. . . . This permission [given to doctors to practice medicine] is the permission to perform a mitzva, to practice medicine *[l'rap'ot]*, and it falls within the category of preserving life.[24]

Medical Treatment Is Permitted in Spite of Medical Uncertainty

Ramban's comments were prompted by a talmudic discussion that explores the view that a son should not medically treat his parent (through bloodletting) for fear of causing harm in the process:

They asked him: What is the law regarding a son's performing a bloodletting for his father?

—Rav Matana said: "You shall love your neighbor as yourself."[25] [Rashi: The Torah only prohibits Jews from doing to their friends acts they would not wish for themselves.]

—Rav Dimi bar Chanania said: "Striking a person . . . striking an animal."[26] Just as striking an animal for medicinal purposes is blameless, so is striking a person for medicinal purposes blameless.

Mar son of Ravina did not permit his son to lance open a blister [bu'ai] lest he should wound him and he would have negligently transgressed a prohibition.

—If so, this is true of another as well!

——Another would have negligently transgressed a prohibition, but a son would negligently transgress a hanging offense.[27]

As an exceptional case, the codified law understands this passage to permit a child to treat a parent when no other person to care for the patient is available and the parent requests the child to act. As a general rule, however, the child should not treat the parent because the legal consequences of a child's error are more strict than those of another.[28] Of this passage Ramban writes:

This is astonishing, for if that were so no expert will involve himself in medical treatment at all, in case he might err [and the patient die] and this should be accounted to him as a negligent performance of what is otherwise a capital offense. Moreover, what does it matter whether it is a son who bloodlets his father, or one who bloodlets his friend?—For in any event it is possible that the patient shall be harmed, for bloodletting involves a variety of dangers! And too: If *we* are concerned regarding the doctor, *the patient* should be concerned *on his own behalf,* for if they treat him with drugs and he ingests them, or with herbal preparations which he drinks, they may have erred regarding diagnosis or treatment, and as a result he has killed himself, for "a physician's mistake is a lethal drug." And so we find the patient himself has entered the realm of risk.

And so it should be said that since permission was given to the doctor to treat, and this is even a commandment imposed by the Merciful One, he should not be concerned at all; for if he treats them as is appropriate, according to his own judgment, his medical treatment is nothing more than a mitzva, that the Merciful One has commanded. . . . [Indeed,] Striking a person for medical treatment is a *mitzva,* that of loving your neighbor as yourself. . . . [29] *You have nothing in medical treatment but danger, that which heals one kills the other.*[30]

Put in another way: Medical uncertainty, unpacked, translates into patient risk; in Ramban's pithy adage, "A physician's mistake is a lethal drug." For Ramban, too, this is a two-sided proposition: Were the physician required to refrain from his or her practice on account of risk, the patient would be required to refrain from seeking medical assistance for that same reason. In fact, the license given to a physician to heal—the license to take risks—is a license held by the patient as well.

Because of this uncertainty, reliable and precise risk-benefit calculations are frequently lacking. The patient (and physician) are left to fall back upon certain presumptions, rules of thumb, which allow (and which may even require) action based upon admittedly incomplete and imperfect knowledge, for "the judge has nothing other than that which his eyes see." The principle that to my mind emerges from these discussions is this: A patient with a lethal illness, a patient whose options are grim, is given relatively free sway to express his or her values in reaching a medical decision. In such cases, there is no definitive answer to the question: "What would a reasonable caretaker do now?"

Rational Action Under Conditions of Uncertainty: Contemporary Dilemmas

The issue raised in this section is far from settled today. Activism on behalf of persons with AIDS has in large part focused around access to experimental treatments, particularly on behalf of persons in a late stage of the disease, who are commonly excluded from clinical trials. The early stage of investigating new cancer drugs (known as "Phase I trials") relies upon volunteers whose cancer has proven untreatable by any established methods.

In both cases, participants are facing very heavy odds that experimental treatment will be of any personal benefit to them—although over time, the progress of clinical medicine, and improved treatments to future patients, very much relies upon such choices. Consider the cancer example. One 1984 study reviewed the results in a very large collection of Phase I studies, which had between them enrolled 1248 subjects. That review found that only two patients (0.16%) achieved total remission and that even when partial responses were counted as benefit, only 2% had been helped. The odds of improvement on Phase I trials are so poor that a special task force of the (U.S.) National Cancer Institute and the Food and Drug Administration has insisted that "information disclosed for Phase I must include a statement about the small possibility of direct benefit to the patient him/herself."[31]

It is tempting, facing such numbers, to conclude that any person who enrolls in such a study must be, at best, self-deluding; at worst, misinformed, by the connivance of clinical investigators who take the stance that when experimenting upon the dying, "anything goes." To say that would, however, be tantamount to saying that it is irrational for patients to make such choices. The sources we have examined suggest to the contrary: There is no such thing as a single "rational response" to such choices; if there were, that rational response would define what is required of the patient as a reasonable caretaker of his or her body. Rather than a single rational response, there are many: It is rational for dying patients to live their last days as though they are living, rather than dying, in a manner fully consistent with how they have lived their lives up until this point—a decision only they can reach, and one that can only be reached after the patient has been fully informed of the nature and consequences of the choice in question.

Allowable Risks 2:
Risking Pain and Life for Quality of Life

The previous section considered health care decisions along a single dimension, time. Persons do, however, value more than length of life; they value quality of life as well. Yet, judgments of quality of life are notoriously subjective. It is structurally difficult for a regimen of duty such as Judaism to accommodate the notion of quality of life when understood as the mere expression of individual patient preference; individual preference, if given an important role, puts a perpetual check upon the demands of duty. Nonetheless, a position on quality of life may be established by means of community reflection and, ultimately, preference.

Jewish Attitudes Toward Pain

It would be impossible, for example, to approach the legal question of quantity and quality of life in Judaism without considering the underlying valuational inquiry into Jewish attitudes toward pain and suffering. It is undeniable that Judaism, in common with many other religious and philosophical traditions, assigned some value to suffering and the positive effects it has—"purifying" the soul and leading persons to repent. In principle, then, the Talmud states that it is a privilege to suffer for seven years rather than to die instantly.[32] Overall, however, the negative aspects of pain were held to outweigh the positive, so that when the suffering rabbi was asked, "Are your torments dear to you?" he responded, "Neither they nor their reward."[33]

More ascetic traditions may see pain as a mixed blessing. It would be more accurate to say that for Judaism pain is, rather, a mixed curse: despite its good points, it is something that one should avoid. A good illustration is found in an oft-quoted incident that occurred while Rabbi lay dying of a painful gastrointestinal illness. (Rabbi Yehuda the Prince, who prepared the Mishna in its final form, was because of his preeminence known simply as "Rabbi.")

On that day when Rabbi's soul rested, the rabbis had decreed a fast, and they prayed for mercy. Moreover they decreed: Anyone who should say, "The soul of Rabbi goes to rest" shall be pierced through with a sword. Rabbi's maidservant went up to the roof, and said: Those Above are seeking Rabbi, and those below are seeking Rabbi; may it be Thy will that those below overpower those Above. When she saw the many times that he went to the bathroom, taking off his phylacteries and setting them down in pain, she said: May it be Thy will that those Above overpower those below. Yet the rabbis sought mercy for him without interruption. She took a jug and flung it from the roof to the ground and their beseechings were interrupted; and so Rabbi's soul rested.[34]

This poignant tale found expression in Jewish law. Ran, using it to explain a difficult talmudic passage, ruled that it is a duty to pray for the death of one who is in great suffering.[35] There can be no doubt that for at least one important strand in Judaism, it is acknowledged that life can be so devoid of quality that death is preferable.

Alleviating Pain as a Permitted Goal of Medicine

A number of practical questions now arise. For example: Is it permissible to undergo risk to life on behalf of alleviating pain? One of the most extensive, recent treatments of this question, by R Eli'ezer Waldenberg, is a useful point of departure:

A person who is dangerously ill, whose doctors have despaired of healing him, and suffers greatly from his illness: Is it permitted to institute sedating injections like morphine, even though they do not heal his illness and even though they may, to the contrary, hasten his death? . . .
   In my humble opinion, it seems that any form of medical intervention, given in the form of pills or injections, that is given by a doctor with the goal of alleviating his great suffering, is permitted to be given to the patient, even though it

harms him and may possibly hasten his death, for it appears that this is included in the principle that the Torah gave permission to the doctor to heal—as Ramban in *Torat Ha'adam* explained, that the reason why the Torah needed to give permission to a doctor to heal is because among medicines there is naught but danger, that which heals one kills the other.[36] If so, here too, in giving morphine injections and so on, even though given solely to quieten suffering, nevertheless it appears that this too falls within the class of medical treatment, for there is nothing worse for a man than pain and great suffering. . . .

Moreover, the questioner writes of a case in which the doctors despaired of healing him of his illness. If so, the permission is even more clear; and support for this is found in the words of Ya'avetz, in *Mor Uketzi'a*,[37] who speaks of the permissibility of an operation for gallstones and kidney stones, which was at his time considered to be dangerous, and the patient nonetheless requests that he be operated upon because he is suffering great pain. In his discussion he hesitates in finding this to be permissible, but writes nonetheless that there is room to grant the patient permission to do as he wishes, since his pains are as grievous for him as death. And there it is spoken of a person who will not die without the operation, for a person does not die of pain. *A fortiori*, we can reason that in this case, where the patient has no chance of surviving [that this is permitted]. . . .

And a third: Reason indicates that pains themselves, when they are grievous, hasten death in some measure—"pangs [anacha] even break half a person's body"[38]—and so therefore it is impossible to say exactly which will hasten death more in this critical condition. . . .

And therefore, a doctor is permitted to supply this [treatment], provided it is not given with the aim and prior intention to hasten death, but is rather given with the aim and intention of alleviating his suffering.[39]

Why May Pain Relief Be Sought Despite Risk?

One difficulty in reading any response to a case—whether the response come from a common-law court or from a theologian—is that of extracting the *ratio decidendi,* the reason the judge expressed for deciding the case in the way that he did. Three separate (or, in principle, separable) reasons are offered here by R Waldenberg:

1. The physician is licensed to treat specifically in order to allow the use of risky medical treatments, and the alleviation of pain is a proper medical goal; therefore, treatment is permitted.
2. In cases in which a patient is dying, risky treatments are certainly permitted.
3. The alleviation of pain may prolong, rather than shorten, life; therefore, it is permitted.

Concentrating upon the first reason, it would follow that the permission to utilize risky methods to alleviate pain applies to any patient. The second reason suggests that clear permission is only present when the patient is dying. The third, by contrast, implies that the permission is only present when the "risky" treatment (as judged by its potential to shorten life) is not absolutely risky; that is, when it is also possible (equally possible?) that the "risky" treatment may prolong rather than shorten life.

When one case judgment combines different factors, pulling in opposed directions, clarification is usually sought by comparing other judgments on different cases, "triangulating" toward greater precision in the reasoning. This will not work when, as here, the confounding factors are common to the situation under discussion:

> Concerning one who has cancer that has disseminated such that the doctors do not even think his life may be prolonged by means of an operation; but who operate nonetheless, primarily to reduce his suffering, as is common in prostate cancer . . . This is permitted, for a patient who is in danger may even undergo an operation to reduce suffering; and it is also logical that he prolongs his life by some small hour through

this, although the doctors are not aware of that. For it is surely logical that two patients who are in danger from the self-same disease, one of whom is suffering while the other of whom is not suffering—that it would be natural for the one without suffering to live a bit longer than the one who is in pain, for great pains themselves shorten life. Therefore, it is certainly permitted to do this.[40]

How much of these responsa is restricted to the facts of the case before them, and how much of what they say is to be generalized to other cases—and how? Consider their handling of the question of pain and survival. I am torn two ways in my reaction to the fact that both of these responsa reject the premise of the question: Asked whether a dangerous treatment may be employed, they respond that the treatment is not dangerous. On the one hand, the statements seem to derive from the "physicalist" approach (see my Introduction), and as such to be irrelevant and even presumptuous. After all, these rabbis were not asked about the permissibility of nondangerous treatments, and they possess neither the education nor the authority to provide scientific conclusions about medical treatments. On the other hand, they point to a fact that is frequently ignored or elided by the questioner. Certainly I have often met with families of incompetent patients who were concerned about the risks associated with pain medication, but who failed to weigh these against the risks associated with pain itself—often, because they were not told of those risks.

The problem posed to R Waldenberg is a good example of this. Morphine is dangerous because the doses that may be required over time (as the patient develops drug tolerance) to suppress pain may suppress the patient's breathing. But morphine also may *improve* a patient's breathing, by alleviating chest pain that causes the patient to take shallow breaths.

Understanding the Rabbinic Responses to the Problem of Pain Relief

This, however, returns us to the problem of generalizing these discussions. Is it only when treatments may prolong as well as shorten life, as in the cases of morphine injection and prostate surgery—or worse yet, in these *particular* cases of morphine and surgery—that risky treatments for pain relief may be attempted? Or do they mean to be asserting, for example, as a scientific matter, that in every case pain relief has the potential to prolong rather than to shorten life?

Considering the interplay of the other factors noted in these and related responsa compounds the difficulties. R Feinstein seemed to join R Waldenberg in ruling that pain relief is an acceptable goal of treatment. Yet R Feinstein had elsewhere stated that "if there are drugs that relieve the pain *and do not shorten even one moment of life* these should be given."[41] This seems to conflict with the inference from Ramban's *Torat Ha'Adam* that reasons that since all treatment involves risk, risk may be faced on behalf of the alleviation of pain.[42] Or should R Feinstein's statement be understood narrowly, as prohibiting those drugs that are given for the sole purpose of shortening life?

Another issue: Does the concept of pain embrace psychological suffering and anguish for these purposes? As we will see in our later discussion of cosmetic surgery, R Waldenberg appears to reject such an extension, while other writers[43] specifically refer to great psychological pain *[sevel nefesh chazak m'od]* as an important consideration.

Relieving Pain: Ethical as Well as Medical Uncertainty

I find no definitive resolution of these issues. In fact, the theme that seems to emerge from the problem of risk and extreme pain is precisely one of uncertainty, ethical as well as medical. In the meantime, how may a responsible caretaker act under these tragic circumstances? There is no retreating to the quietist principle "sit and do not act," if indeed the imperative to treat encompasses the imperative to relieve pain.

The issue of action under uncertainty appears to be the leitmotif in the following excerpt from R Feinstein's writings. He is asked whether there is an obligation to treat a patient who is in great pain with the aim of prolonging the patient's life. In the absence of any definitive precedent on this question, he decides upon a procedural rather than a substantive solution; in cases when we do not know what to decide, all we can determine is who should decide.

If it is impossible to heal a patient but to give him drugs to prolong his life as he is, in his disease and pain, for many years, or
even to live an ordinary life span such as people live today, is
there an obligation to heal him? . . . In a case when he suffers
and there is no known medical method to alleviate his suffering, such that a person even prefers to die than to live a life of
such pain . . . it seems on its face logical that there is no obligation to treat such a patient when he doesn't wish treatments
that prolong his painful existence. And generally, when it is not
possible to know the views of the patient, we can assume that
the patient does not want it and there is no obligation to treat
him; but in the overwhelming majority of cases the patient has
relatives, even a father or mother or brothers etc. who involve
themselves in the patient's treatment, and in law this burden is
theirs. . . . [Concerning] whether there should be a distinction
between fleeting life and lasting life, when a person cannot have
his pain alleviated but can only have his life prolonged with its
present suffering . . . there does not indeed seem any reason for
a distinction; and through general reasoning it seems just to the
contrary [but, since there is no talmudic precedent on this
question it is uncertain] so that if such a case should, Heaven
forbid, arise, we do not know how to rule. Therefore, the matter is given over to the view of the patient; and if a minor, to
the view of his father, mother, brothers, etc., for upon them lies
this burden, until the law is clearly established.[44]

The procedural solution suggested here is that used so commonly
by contemporary bioethics. But in Judaism this procedural approach
is the last, rather than the first, resort. It is an admission of failure—
albeit perhaps necessary failure—to answer the personal ethical question: How should a reasonable caretaker act under the pressure of
extreme pain?

Pain Relief in Extremis: Limits of Precedent and of Logic

R Feinstein had no answer to whether a patient in intractable pain
should undergo treatment to prolong his life. He could find no prece-

dent on this question from within talmudic discourse or from subsequent commentators, theologians, and jurists. But why was there no precedent? The reason is that this dilemma is itself the product of medical progress, which has come very far, but not far enough. Patients with astonishing damage, with devastating disease, can have their lives prolonged, sometimes indefinitely, by the use of medical technology and expertise. But our ability to sustain life is often far in advance of our ability to eliminate pain and suffering.

In the times of the Talmud, and for centuries thereafter—indeed, until quite recently—when the pain was bad enough and damage serious enough, a person would necessarily die. Not so today. R Feinstein's failure to find a precedent reflects the fact that modern medicine has, as an unwanted side effect, innovated the heights and depths of pain and suffering that a person can undergo and survive. Within rabbinic literature, the paradigm cases for maximal suffering are found in the tale of the ten rabbinic martyrs,[45] put to death by the Romans for the crime of teaching Torah. The tortures they suffered were terrible indeed, but I believe the potential of a modern hospital to inflict pain and suffering exceeds that of any Roman master of torture, because in a hospital death is not a reliable and timely deliverance. Rabbi Akiva had his skin flayed from him with iron combs and died. A burning victim today can have his skin flayed as well—debridement of dead and burned skin—again and again and again and can survive being skinned over a major portion of his body, the infections that will follow, and many surgical grafting procedures thereafter. Rabbi Chanina ben Teradyon, we are told, was burned alive; the torture master had him wrapped in wet cloth to prolong his anguish; and he died. We can go the Romans several better than that today—when our patients are burning up alive with fever, for example. Their ending is not in all cases as merciful as was his.

There is a second reason why R Feinstein found no answer. Even when there is no precedent, logic would ordinarily show the way. But in this case, he found, logic failed him. I do not believe R Feinstein is alone in finding that logic is an insufficient guide in these extreme cases, in which it seems that whatever you will do will be wrong. The following consultation note illustrates the point.

ETHICS DISCUSSION: SNOWING IN OCTOBER

Mrs. X is a sixty-six-year-old woman with advanced and intractable esophageal cancer. The issue concerned her medical management during this final admission and terminal phase. This note is prepared following a discussion with the attending physician responsible for her basic hospital care, Dr. D, on October 2, that was followed up by a meeting of the medical and nursing team in that unit at 2 PM, on October 6. The patient had expired in the interim. It was felt that the scheduled meeting remained important because of the issues and emotions raised by the care of Mrs. X.

The patient had been cared for by a family physician, Dr. E, and in a later stage by Dr. C, a medical oncologist. Her cancer had not responded to standard treatment, and she opted for treatment on an experimental protocol, which itself failed to arrest the progression of her disease and caused substantial side effects.

In discussions with all three doctors mentioned above, Mrs. X and her husband had expressed the desire that the doctors "provide her with euthanasia," i.e., kill her. The primary motivation for this was anguish, suffering at her state and future prospects, rather than pain itself (although her pain and nausea may not have been fully controlled at all times). She was an active woman who had in the later stages of her illness consented to treatment and retreatment more in the hope of regaining function and some mobility than for cure. She could not bear being bedridden, and she had asked that her friends not come and visit her because she did not want them to see her in this state.

She was told that euthanasia was not something any of the staff were prepared to consider. At one point, though, her doctor offered to discharge her home with a month's supply of pain medication. That would have permitted her and her husband to arrange her suicide, but this was declined: They wanted her to remain in hospital.

As a result of her suffering, she said, the only time that she is comfortable is when she is sleeping, and not ruminating on her condition. An alternative possibility was offered to her by Dr. C, the oncologist: If nothing else would help, she could be given enough pain medication so that she would sleep continuously, i.e., be "snowed under." This was the choice she settled upon, with the agreement of her husband. Her children were aware of the arrangement, and acquiesced as well.

A period of more than a week was required to find the right dosages and combinations of medications to achieve the desired result. Dr. D was left with this task and was frustrated and rebuffed in efforts to get some advice about this from anesthesiology and palliative care specialists in other city hospitals. In the interim period Mrs. X, in times of lucidity, repeated her desire that this be done. Even after this medically induced state of coma was achieved, however, her husband continued to insist that she was suffering and should be euthanized. After seven to ten days or so of being snowed under, Mrs. X did expire.

The discussions were intended to review and explore this case and its associated issues and feelings. I had been told that several nurses were uncomfortable with the course of action chosen, although at the meeting, attended by many nurses, only one admitted to feeling this way. (She had asked not to be assigned to this patient, and her wishes were respected.)

Nevertheless, many of those affected, doctors and nurses alike, expressed discomfort or feelings of failure about the course of events. These feelings were reinforced by the negative feedback experienced when consults on the treatment regimen were requested. I experienced this myself, in the reaction I had gotten from a colleague when discussing this case who believed the case had been mishandled. There should have been a better palliative resolution, in his view; he suggested that counseling and a psychiatric consultation should have been pursued. He pointed to the ambiguity of decisions made by Mrs. X and her husband, as in their declining the opportunity to be discharged home. Another example: While asleep most of the time due to the medication, when awake, Mrs. X did eat at mealtimes.

The question of whether "there was anything further that could have been tried" was discussed at some length. The question of psychiatric involvement and counseling had not been raised with the patient, but all who know her were certain she would have rejected this: She was not crazy, and her reaction was a reasonable and human one to terrible life circumstances. It was also felt that even had she consented, psychiatry had nothing useful to offer her.

That apart, there were other things that could have been tried—as there always are—but the question is: Should they have been? She knew how she wanted to spend the very limited time she had remaining, and it was within the power of her doctors to supply that. This was not a case in which we immediately agreed to a patient's request to be "snowed under," simply because that is how the patient wanted to be treated. Here we were faced with a lucid woman who had tried standard and even experimental treatment, failed both, and was at the end of her rope. Will all her time remaining be spent in futile, paternalistic efforts at finding a medical or psychiatric magic bullet that will reconcile her to a brief, bedridden existence?

Everybody agreed with the concept that the patient, as a person, needs to be treated under concepts of total pain burden that do not give more significance to "physical pain" than to psychological anguish, and yet, paradoxically, everyone would have felt more comfortable in reaching this decision to snow the patient under if it were the only way to control physical pain. I suggested, and some agreed, that it would be wrong to give in to this ill-grounded, medicalizing prejudice.

A consensus was reached at the second meeting that the course of action was proper under the circumstances. Still, we need to realize in advance that anytime such a decision is reached it can always be second-guessed and will always carry with it a burden of guilt: While a patient's request to be snowed under is resisted and alternatives are pursued, we are wrong in inflicting unwanted treatment; once a patient's wishes are respected, we can always say that something further should have been tried. It was because no resolution is fully satisfactory that the outside consultations were so negative, rather than because the particular resolution reached was wrong. Finally, and for the same reason, it was agreed that staff who disagree with this form of management should have their wishes to be relieved of looking after the patient respected if at all possible.

I do not mean to suggest, in quoting this case, that any of the rabbinic authorities whose views were described here would have validated its resolution. I have not seen the issue discussed and am uncertain how they would react. Certainly, however, the extreme difficulty that all of us felt in reaching and discussing this resolution seems to me to echo in the last-quoted excerpt of R Feinstein.

Pain and Wounding; Pain Along a Continuum

Pain is, of course, not merely the absence of pleasure, but the absence of pleasure is, or can be, a component of pain. The next talmudic passage delves into this point regarding the reasonable caretaker's responsibility to the self in the course of clarifying a statement that persons are forbidden to wound themselves. In analyzing proposed foundations for the rule against self-wounding—two of which are rejected, while the third seems to be accepted—the Talmud at the same time implicitly states parameters for the trade-offs that a reasonable caretaker may undertake:[46]

> What is the source for the teaching that rules that a person is not permitted to wound himself?
> We might say this one: "It was taught: "Yet your blood from your own souls I shall seek"[47]—R El'azar said, from your souls I shall seek your own blood."
> —But perhaps killing is different.

The reasonable caretaker is enjoined against wounding himself (chavala), and its accompanying suffering. The prohibition is important in the context of considering when consent to surgery, or even to invasive medical treatments, is consistent with the responsibilities of the reasonable caretaker. The first proposal asks us to derive the prohibition against self-wounding as a corollary deriving from a biblical verse understood to prohibit suicide. This proposal is, however, rejected. "Killing is different" from "wounding" and pain; the laws regarding quantity of life are incommensurate with those regarding quality of life. A second proposal is therefore offered:

> Perhaps, from this teaching: "It was taught, 'We tear garments on behalf of the dead [i.e. as a sign of mourning], and this practice is not among the [forbidden, idolatrous] ways of the Amorites'; R El'azar said, 'I had heard that one who tears his garments on behalf of the dead too much is punished by flogging on account of the prohibition against wastefulness [*bal tashchit*],—how much more so regarding [harming] the body!'"
> —Yet perhaps clothes are different, for they involve financial loss, for they do not repair themselves; as in the passage, "R Yochanan used to call his clothes 'That which gives me honor'; and R Chisda: When he would walk among thorns, he would lift his clothes, as he said, 'One [my skin] will be made whole, the other [my clothes] would not be made whole.'"

The second proposal reasons from the general prohibition against causing wanton damage to a specific prohibition against causing damage to one's own physical self. This too is set aside, by citing the curious story of R Chisda, who chose to let his skin be scratched rather than let his garments be torn, with the accompanying wastage and financial loss.

In rejecting the proposal, the Talmud in fact lifts the analytic divide often erected between risk-benefit analysis, which only considers harms to persons themselves, and cost-benefit analysis, which at least includes (if indeed it does not restrict itself to) financial considerations. This passage, and its tale of R Chisda, stands as a source for the proposition that at least at certain minimal levels of harm, the responsible caretaker is permitted to factor into decision making the financial implications of choice. Having established that irreparable financial harm may outweigh minor physical wounds that will be self-healing, it is impossible to derive a prohibition against the latter from the former.[48]

A third proposal is therefore attempted. It derives from the Biblical laws of a Nazirite [nazir], one who has voluntarily taken an ascetic vow to refrain from some of the ordinary pleasures of life, for example, drinking wine or grooming his hair. Following the Naziritic period, this person is required to bring a sacrifice at the Temple, a sin-offering. The question is: What is the sin which he has committed that requires this act of atonement?

> Rather, this teaching is in accord with the following: "We learned: R El'azar Hakappar Berabbi said, What is taught by saying, 'He shall be atoned in that he had sinned against the soul'—[49] Against what soul had he sinned? Rather: He had caused himself pain by [withholding] wine. The argument holds *a fortiori:* If one who caused himself pain only by withholding wine from himself is called a sinner, how much more so someone who harms himself in another way!"

The prohibition against self-wounding is at last grounded upon the proposition that the reasonable caretaker should not deny himself benefit in the world without adequate motivation. Elsewhere, the lesson is put this way: "In the future [i.e., in the time of final judgment], every man will be called to account for everything he had seen and not eaten,"[50] that is, every lawful pleasure that he had denied himself.

To sum up: In general, the active causing of wounding and its accompanying pain is judged along a continuum that extends to the withholding of allowable pleasures. Suffering a wound to be caused, or even causing it oneself, is permitted to the person exercising responsible stewardship, provided this is done for a proportional cause, as in the case of R Chisda; contrariwise, the denial to oneself of a pleasure is impermissible if inadequately motivated. Yet at the limit there is a break in this continuum: "Killing is different," and the ordinary weighing and counterbalancing of considerations that suffices when judging actions that involve self-wounding *[chavala]* and suffering *[tza'ar]* do not apply in the same way when considering serious risk to life *[sakana].*[51]

Considerations of Risk and Wounding: The Case of Cosmetic Surgery

These principles of responsible judgment are illustrated well in some of the rabbinic literature that has appeared concerning the permissibility of cosmetic surgery. The range of views has been summed up by Prof. Abraham S. Abraham[52] as follows:

Plastic surgery: There exists a difference of opinion whether such an operation is permitted, with the goal of beauty for the sake of marriage or household harmony: Some permit it[53] and some forbid it.[54] R Jakobovitz writes[55] that "even if such an operation is not permitted, particularly for males, there is room to permit it if the disfigurement had been caused by an accident or illness, or when it may cause a major depression, or when without it it is impossible for him to find appropriate employment—this truly implicates his livelihood and the financial support of his household."

The issues at stake in the argument may be discerned by examining the view of one of the opponents of cosmetic surgery; as will appear, his rejection is at best equivocal:

Regarding plastic surgery, done to repair or improve appearance or some bodily member that were deviant or harmed in an accident or from birth: Is it permitted to perform such an operation, when there is no obvious need for it, and it is simply done for the sake of beauty; since, in such an operation, we find aspects of both self-wounding, and even danger?
. . . Regarding the reason of self-wounding, we see from Rambam[56] that apparently only acts done in in a manner designed to humiliate *[derekh bizayon]* are prohibited [and it

may be argued that cosmetic surgery does not fall within this category]. . . .

But regarding danger there remains a serious problem . . . and although my honored correspondent presented a powerful logical argument, that certainly he does this out of necessity, and has some worry or mental derangement [teruf da'at] caused by his situation and appearance which he wishes to alter by the operation, so that one may say he is considered amongst the class of those who are ill—yet nonetheless he is not in the class of an ill person who is in danger; and the question requires further deliberation.[57]

This author appears to be dealing with a clear case of cosmetic surgery, "done for the sake of beauty" alone, rather than with the broader class of plastic surgery that is performed for functional as well as aesthetic reasons. The issue resolves itself into two questions. First: Is it consistent with the task of a reasonable caretaker to undergo self-wounding and its accompanying pain [chavala and tza'ar] on behalf of the promised improvement of appearance? Second: Is he allowed to undergo risk toward this end?

The first question is resolved in the affirmative. Consistent with the talmudic passage discussed here, a person is permitted to choose to undergo a degree of self-wounding and pain on behalf of that which he or she judges to be a greater good. The author adverts to Rambam's discussion of the general prohibition of wounding, that is, when wounding is in itself and necessarily prohibited. There exist in fact two texts of Rambam on this that qualify, in different ways, the general prohibition. According to one, wounding that is done in a humiliating manner [derekh bizayon] is prohibited; according to another, wounding done in a belligerent manner [derekh nitzayon] is prohibited. Whichever text is chosen, wounding done or allowed on behalf of a proportional benefit has not been per se prohibited. (There will, of course, be differing opinions as to what shall count as a proportional reason. R Moshe Feinstein, in his unequivocally permissive responsum, dealt with a woman seeking self-beautification on behalf of improving her prospects for marriage.)[58]

The second question, regarding the risk associated with surgery, is the sticking point, for "Killing is different." The author of *Minchat Yitzchak* leaves this question undecided. It is undeniable that the person seeking cosmetic surgery may be suffering greatly from his appearance; indeed, *Tosfot*[59] had stated that there is no greater pain than that suffered by one who is embarrassed to go out among people. But while such considerations can override the prohibition against self-wounding, may they override that against endangering life itself? Is the person seeking surgery so distraught that he may be considered to be suffering from a dangerous disease?

It appears that this question of risk is that which divides the other writers on cosmetic surgery. R Waldenberg, who unequivocally prohibits cosmetic surgery,[60] rests his case upon the view of Ramban in *Torat Ha'adam,* who had stated that every single medical intervention involves risk and therefore specific permission had to be supplied to the physician to engage in medicine. This permission, in his view, does not extend to interventions done for cosmetic rather than medical reasons. R Waldenberg does, however, discuss at some length why *chavala* prohibits such surgery as well and denigrates the intent of one seeking, by such surgery, to improve upon the wisdom of his or her Maker. By contrast, R Feinstein, who unequivocally permits cosmetic surgery, does not raise the question of risk in his responsum at all. It may be that what stands between them is a question that will be discussed in a later section, namely: Is there a level of risk that is so low that it may be disregarded by the reasonably conscientious caretaker? If so, where do we locate that level? For, turning to the question of risks that are allowed on behalf of functioning, there is indirect evidence that R Feinstein holds that the lowest common denominator of surgical risk, the risks that necessarily accompany any surgery (e.g., postoperative infection, complications of anesthesia) are not great enough to be considered even "doubtful risk" *[ch'shash sakana].*[61]

The Assumption of Risk and Social Functioning

In cases of cosmetic surgery, it had seemed possible that whereas pain and wounding may be permissible toward this end, serious risk to life is not. Such a stance is consistent with an extremely conservative reading of the idea that the person is charged with responsible caretaking of the body and with the bias for life and safety noted at the beginning of this chapter.

But is it then the case that such serious risks to life may only be voluntarily assumed on behalf of a chance of a prolongation of life itself, as is done by the dangerously ill who agree to surgery? This surely cannot be true, as R Ya'akov Ettlinger, a German authority from the nineteenth century, notes:

> How could it be permissible to travel over the sea, or go forth to travel in the desert?—these acts that are among those for which one who has been preserved must [subsequently] praise and thank [G-d]. How could it be permissible from the outset to enter such danger, thereby transgressing "you shall carefully guard your souls."[62]

A special prayer of thanksgiving had been composed to be recited by those who have been delivered from situations of great danger. When must this blessing be recited? Some of the paradigm cases include situations in which danger was forced upon the victim, for example, one who recovered from a serious illness or one who was released from prison. Other such cases involve dangers that typically have been voluntarily assumed, including those presented here: those who cross the sea or travel over the desert. These feats, so commonplace today, were the source of extremely serious danger during the time of the Talmud and for over a millennium thereafter. How was it permissible for persons to assume such serious risks?[63]

R Ettlinger innovates the following approach to resolve this problem:

> And in my humble opinion, the rabbinic principle that nothing can withstand the requirement to protect life, and further that in matters of protection of life we do not follow the majority, underlies those specific cases where there is a definite danger to life before us, for example, when a wall has fallen upon someone. In those cases, we fret even for the minority of

a minority [i.e., an insignificant chance that by intervening we may preserve the victim's life]. But in those cases when there is at present no threat to life, but one may fret regarding such a threat that may eventually occur, we do follow the majority, just as in other cases of potential transgressions.[64]

This radical view, while noted (if not adopted) by later authorities, is logically hard to follow. R Ettlinger seems to be saying that for present danger, the smallest chance must govern; for danger that has yet to eventuate, any risk of death up to the 50% level is morally acceptable. Logically, when do we say that danger is present, when that it has yet to eventuate? Do you step into danger when you step into a boat, into a boat planning to go where none has gone before, or where many have gone but from which just over half have returned? into a seaworthy boat, into a boat that will almost certainly spring a leak but which is dry at the moment, into a boat that is already leaking but has not yet foundered, whose captain tells you that there is a "better than even" chance that it will stay afloat?

As a practical matter, also, this view is not acceptable. I have heard prudence caricatured by the fool's saying, "Why worry until something bad happens?" R Ettlinger's responsum implies that this is an acceptable stance for the reasonable caretaker, but it is of course antithetical to the foresight and caution that is expected of a caretaker.

Acceptable Risk and Occupational Exposure

There is, fortunately, a much better approach to the problem R Ettlinger poses. A person does not act irresponsibly in exposing himself or herself to occupational danger, to risk undertaken on behalf of livelihood; and, to some extent, the allowable level of danger may rise according to the desperateness of one's economic straits. One source for this principle arises in a discussion of the biblical prohibition against delaying the wages of a worker:

"To that he hands over his soul":[65] Why does this man ascend a ladder, or suspend himself from a tree, handing himself over to death? For nothing other than his wages.[66]

This principle of allowable risk is applied by R Yechezkel Landau, an eighteenth-century rabbi from Poland, known eponymously for his collection of responsa, *Nod'a BiYehuda:*

> The source of his question: One man whom G-d had blessed with a large inheritance, within which are villages and forests; and in those forests swarm all manner of wild animals. Is he permitted to go himself and shoot with a rifle *[kane s'refa]* for hunting, or is such prohibited to a Jew? . . . Now I say: There is even a prohibition here, for all of those who involve themselves in this must enter the forests and face great dangers where wild animals gather, and the Merciful One had said, "take great care of your souls." . . . How then can a Jew enter a place where wild animals gather? Yet nevertheless, one who is poor and does this for his subsistence *[michyato]* has been permitted to do so by the Torah, *as is true of all those merchants who cross the sea;* for whatever is done for the sake of his subsistence and occupation *[parnasato]*—he has no choice. . . . But one whose basic intention is not for his subsistence, but who exposes himself to danger and faces the place where wild animals gather out of the lust of his heart, violates a prohibition.[67]

In an almost off-hand, quite elegant way, R Landau resolves the question posed by R Ettlinger. One who "crosses the sea" may do so because he is a merchant and this is his job, although he could not have done so out of personal preference, for example, as recreation.

How much risk is permitted, on behalf of how much gain?[68] R Landau issues his ruling on behalf of a "poor person" who "has no choice"; but these words should not, I think, be taken too literally. The responsum extends permission not only to those who need to take risks on behalf of having food to eat—bare subsistence, *michya*—but also to those whose occupation, *parnasa,* entails risk. The dignity and value that Jewish sources have traditionally attributed to labor may be the underlying basis for this extended permission. The poor person, after all, has the choice of being supported by others: in eighteenth-century Poland, by the communal provision to the poor of foodstuffs *[tamchui]* and money for the necessities of life *[kupa]*; in twentieth-century America, by welfare and food stamps, if not by a less risky occupation. (The contemporary American authority, R Moshe Feinstein stated that a person is permitted to make his livelihood by engaging in dangerous sports.)[69]

Nor can the principle be limited to occupational requirements, or other financial circumstances. Persons are more than just economic units. Rather, it must be understood as encompassing both occupations and any other important social role (e.g., marriage, filial duty) that person occupies or plans to occupy.[70]

Medical Risk and Social Roles as a Continuing Issue

These questions continue to arise today, in debates over occupational risk and the existence (and propriety) of associated "risk premiums," hazard pay provided to those who undertake dangerous tasks.[71] And new ones loom on the horizon, as in the issue of whether persons at extremely high occupational risk of contracting AIDS should be compensated for this risk over and above compensation for the work they perform.[72]

In medical jurisprudence, too, we find recognition that such occupational concerns are legitimate on the part of patients. The landmark Canadian case on informed consent to medical treatment, *Reibl v. Hughes,*[73] turned on just such an issue. The patient, Mr. Reibl, had not been informed of the risk that a recommended surgical procedure (carotid endarterectomy) carried with it a substantial risk of surgically induced stroke resulting in death (estimated at 4%) or permanent paralysis (estimated at a further 10%). There was no dispute that the procedure was indicated; without it, Mr. Reibl faced a high risk of stroke, which would grow year by year. The average reasonable person would choose immediate surgery, the court found, trading in the higher risks of stroke caused by a narrowing of an artery for the lower risks of stroke caused by surgery itself. But Mr. Reibl was not an "average, reasonable patient," as the surgeon was or should have been aware. A long-time employee of a large firm, he would have kept working for the brief period pending until his pension benefits were assured, and so delayed his surgery. In Canadian law, the concept of an "average, reasonable patient" cannot be understood without considering that person's specific life plans, including economic circumstances. In Jewish law, the concept of an "average, reasonable caretaker" is similarly socially conditioned.

(The difference between the Canadian regime of rights and the Jewish regime of duty should, however, be noted. In Canada, if some fact is potentially relevant to the decision a reasonable patient might reach, the patient has a right to be informed of this. In Judaism, if some fact is potentially relevant to the decision of a reasonable caretaker, the patient has a duty to consider that fact and take it into account. In either case, the doctor has a duty to disclose the information; in the case of Canadian law, that duty is secondary to the patient's right; in Jewish law, the doctor's duty is secondary to the patient's duty.)

These principles, however, leave open some difficult questions. Social circumstances are ill-defined and represent a wild card in decision making. We have grown used to a world in which the traditional sources of risks—travel, food, work, childbirth, etc.—have been driven, through technological advance and vigorous government regulation, to unprecedentedly low levels; in some cases, one-hundredth or even one-thousandth what they had been in the time of *Nod'a BiYehuda*. It is easy to imagine that the level of risk accepted without comment two hundred years ago would be ruled completely unacceptable today on behalf of anything other than the most urgent activities. The principle of allowed occupational risk introduces us to the problem of the social relativity of allowable risk, which we must now confront directly.

Allowable Risks 3:
The Threshold of Risk: "G-d Protects Fools"

Trade-offs of Pain, Risk, and Finances

Patients who have health insurance (whether private or governmental) frequently face the choice of accepting the treatment covered by insurance or directly paying for a superior quality of treatment. The superior treatment in question might be a drug or diagnostic test with fewer side effects, a prosthetic device that is more adaptive and comfortable, or the opportunity to have an immediate operation rather than languishing on a waiting list. Many of these choices involve a clear and immediate advantage to the patient: an antibiotic that doesn't cause diarrhea, a prosthetic that provides a better range of movement. Often, in addition, there is an extremely small increment of safety that can be purchased by buying out of the system. A patient who chooses to pay for immediate surgery rather than waiting for three months is not only spared the anguish of waiting but also avoids the possibility that in the interim his condition may worsen, or even become inoperable. Is the patient who attempts to act as a reasonable caretaker obliged to buy his way out of the system in search of better treatment?

Recast in Jewish terms, we may say, the choice to forgo insurance benefits and pay out of pocket for a superior therapeutic modality often involves a substantial benefit along the dimension of pain *[tza'ar]*, and sometimes an extremely small advantage along that of danger *[sakana]*. Are both choices consistent with the duties a caretaker possesses regarding his or her body?

As regards a patient's decision about *tza'ar*, it is arguable that only the patient knows enough about his own pain, and his own need for, or alternative uses for, the money (i.e., the "opportunity costs" of the decision), to judge properly. We will pursue later the reasons for considering that only patients can judge their own pain, and the implications that follow. Given that fact, however, the personal nature of a risk-benefit (or cost-benefit) calculation is evident, and can in fact commonly be straightforwardly inferred from the choice the patient actually makes. (The assumption is the same as that expressed in the economists' phrase, "revealed preference.") R Moshe Feinstein provides a good illustration of this in discussing the decision a Nazirite has reached to take that vow and to deny himself wine:

> We must say that when one denies himself [the pleasure associated with] the drinking of wine on behalf of some other advantage he is not considered to have caused himself any *tza'ar*, since his pleasure from the advantage outweighs his pain; for

when he drinks and forgoes the advantage he will have still more pain from the fact that he has lost the advantage that he would gain by not drinking at all—for all of his pain from being denied the wine derives from his appetite for it, and he has a greater appetite for the advantage.[74]

In other words, pain, *tza'ar*, is a bottom-line judgment for the patient to make. If short-term pain is outweighed by long-term gain, the patient may choose the former (and, in some cases, might be obliged to choose the former; although, by the nature of things, nobody other than G-d will know the patient has violated his duty). A patient's decision to accept an inferior prosthetic, painful and even debilitating side effects, and so on, rather than pay to avoid these harms, would seem to be his to make. (And because it is his to make, it is absolutely imperative that the patient be provided with sufficient information to arrive at a personal decision, consistent with his own values.)

But, may the judgment of risk, *sakana*, be left up to the patient as well? Or, in cases of tiny but genuine risk, as may occur in delayed surgery, is the patient required, as a reasonable caretaker, to spare no expense? Two sets of sources bear on this question, each leading to the conclusion that a person is permitted to ignore known but highly improbable risks.

First Approach: Discounting Highly Improbable Risk

One line of thought simply denies the legal relevance of very remote possibilities. The *locus classicus* for this position is found in an oft-quoted responsum of R Moshe Sofer, dealing with a government decree that prohibited the declaration of death until a physician had examined the body and found physical signs of decomposition. This decree conflicts with the position of Jewish law that requires the body be buried as expeditiously as possible. As such, the *Chatam Sofer* writes, the decree must be resisted, and death should continue to be declared on the basis of proof that the person had ceased to breathe; this despite the fact that some few people may erroneously be declared to be dead by this criterion (as indeed had happened in one case described in the Talmud):

The truth will show us its path, for this [talmudic case] is just a random occurrence from those unlikely events that happen once in a thousand years, that one should arise after he had fallen down and stopped breathing. . . . This isn't even a minority of a minority; like the [miracle story told of a Jewish Rip van Winkle, the] occurrence of Choni the circle-drawer, who slept for seventy years. . . . For thus did the Giver of the Torah command us, blessed be His name: that we should rule according to the usual case. Just as we eat meat: Even though it occurs that a minority of cases of animals are [unbeknownst to us] *trefa* [ritually unfit for consumption], we have nevertheless eaten with permission, for He did not ask of us anything more than that we eat from the majority.[75]

A similar view is expressed by R Tzvi Hirsch Chayes:[76] "Even though regarding protection of life we do not follow the majority, nevertheless since the exceptions are one in millions, for such a minority of a minority we do not take concern"; and, by R Chaim Yosef David 'Azula'i: "If it should happen once in tens of thousands of times that he is alive, we are not burdened by even a speck of prohibition."[77]

The principle—that even grave risks (literally "grave": the discussions devolve around burial in error) may be ignored if highly improbable—is clear enough, although quantitatively ill-defined (one in "millions"? "tens of thousands"?). We can ask, from the point of view of risk-benefit reasoning, whether this principle is rationally defensible. Why should we ignore highly unlikely events, rather than simply weight them very lightly? Why not "play it safe," "err on the side of life"? I find it suggestive that these very extreme cases reveal that the Jewish regime of duty rarely, if ever, allows one to retreat to such a reflexive, unconsidered, conservative stance. Even here there is no way to play it safe, for delayed burial itself—the ultimate "error on the side of life"—is associated with harm.[78]

Second Approach: The Allowable Risks of Everyday Life

The second set of sources have even broader implications. They take off from several talmudic discussions of practices considered risky.

For example, the Babylonian Talmud[79] discusses the question of blood-letting prior to the Sabbath, considered to be a risky time for this practice because of accepted astrological considerations.[80] The Talmud states that the practice is permitted despite this risk, reasoning that, "Once many have trampled upon it, 'G-d protects fools.'"[81] (Rashi explains there that Friday had become a popular time for "prophylactic" bloodletting, to prepare for the large Sabbath meals by this procedure, believed to assist digestion.) The same phrase is invoked on numerous other occasions as justification for accepted risky practices.[82]

The vicissitudes this principle experienced over the succeeding centuries of rabbinic discussion reflect tensions arising from the principle's rationale. The verse appealed to by the principle was "G-d protects fools." The term for fools used here is p'ta'im, the plural form of peti, a form of incompetence discussed earlier (see Section 3) in which a person is intellectually incapable of reliably "guarding" the self. The verse appears in this context: The Psalmist sings of having been endangered, possibly by illness, and rescued by G-d's grace. He praises G-d for His salvation and brings sacrifices of thanksgiving.

The normative implications of the verse are unclear, particularly when juxtaposed with a seemingly opposing principle that requires that people not rely upon G-d's grace (in the form of a miracle) to protect them from danger.[83] Does the verse then teach us that anyone may rely upon G-d's assistance? When, and under what circumstances? Does it teach that it is in fact particularly praiseworthy to have this depth of faith in G-d? Or does it perhaps simply mean that if one had foolishly—and wrongly—failed in one's duty of self-protection and been saved from the consequences of one's folly, that praise is due to G-d?

These tensions and ambiguities have resulted in a series of inconsistent rabbinic reactions to the principle. One view has it that such faith in G-d is not simply praiseworthy (still less, simply optional) but in fact obligatory. It follows for this view that because the Talmud states of some risky practice x, "Once many have trampled upon it, 'G-d protects fools,'" it would be a culpable absence of faith to fail to do x.[84] In another view, this kind of faith is praiseworthy but is the prerogative of the exceedingly pious; it is presumptuous for ordinary folk to rely upon G-d's protection in this way.[85] At the other extreme, one view has it that one may never rely upon this principle a priori; after the fact, when risk has already been incurred, it may be that the damage will be mitigated because of the principle.[86]

This ambivalence is reflected in diverging views regarding the scope of the principle as well: Is it to be invoked narrowly or broadly? One view has it that the principle is solely restricted to the cases presented in the Talmud; other dangers, new risks, may not be faced in reliance upon the principle. (It appears that the motivation for narrowing the principle's scope is to permit the taking of precautions against these new dangers, rather than to prohibit the new occasions for danger.)[87] But many other rabbis have broadened its scope and have ruled that various new allegations of risky conduct need not be heeded because "G-d protects fools."[88]

"G-d Protects Fools": One Approach

It is impossible to reconcile all the different opinions on this principle.[89] Instead, I want to focus upon one reading of this principle, its rationale, and its scope. This view understands the principle as granting the reasonable caretaker permission to engage in activities that the general population have come to accept despite the (relatively improbable) risks they might entail.

Here is an example of how this understanding was applied. The question raised: A hospital wishes to use medical monitors with alarms as a substitute for frequent checks by medical attendants:

> In addition to what has been said, we found that our Sages of blessed memory said about the performance of an act that is associated with the possibility of danger, and yet [one which] many are accustomed not to hesitate to do—although it is impossible to say of it that such is literally the custom of the entire world—nevertheless, they have ruled on such cases by deciding: Now that many have trampled upon it "G-d protects the simple." That is to say, even something that had previously been the cause of concern because of its associated danger, something people were careful to avoid, yet since

afterwards many resolved not to be concerned about this and to do it, is no longer considered in the class of dangers that we rule must not be performed, provided the danger is not very clear; rather, we may rely upon Heavenly mercy.[90]

Two qualifications must be satisfied for the risky activity to be permissible: First, the risk must be improbable;[91] second, it must be an activity widely (although not necessarily universally) engaged in, without its participants particularly noticing the minor risk to which they are exposed.[92] By contrast, as R Basil Herring notes, "What would be forbidden are acts that are generally perceived as dangerous, and which most people are careful to avoid. . . . Implicit in this approach is the recognition of the possibility of change, in accordance with social trends and habits."[93]

This particular view of the principle seems to me to be supported by a close reading of the talmudic expression. The beginning of the talmudic phrase "once the many have trampled upon it" serves to define its scope. The term used, "trample"—its Hebrew root, *DSH*—is a verb that has the specific implication of incidental, offhand damage, stepping on something while barely noticing that fact,[94] and came to refer to the kind of "background noise" to which one is so accustomed that it is no longer noticed.[95] Because some risk is so low, says this principle, that people scarcely notice it at all, we need not take precautions against it; but may instead act as does the fool, the *peti,* a person who, because of intellectual incapacity, does not guard himself. Or in other words: At this point, because risks have been *accepted* (as a matter of social reality) they have become *acceptable* (as a matter of Jewish law and personal morality).

Thresholds of Risk:
An Inescapable Necessity of Ethics and Policy

Read in this way, the principle reflects a Jewish response to a problem faced by every modern Western government: the need to establish a threshold of risk, a point at which risk is so improbable that it may be allowed or even ignored by public policy and regulation.[96]

Scientific and technological advances have inexorably increased our knowledge of risks and factors that create risk. Forty years ago, for example, analytic chemists could scarcely detect the presence of a chemical agent found at one part in one million—roughly equivalent to one crystal of salt in a four-ounce jar of sugar. Substances thirty years later could be detected at a level of one part in a trillion—one crystal of salt in one of one million such jars.[97] Now imagine that that crystal of "salt" has been shown to be a potential carcinogen.

Once extraordinarily unlikely risks are contemplated and infinitesimal amounts of agents that might conceivably produce some risk (however unlikely) become measurable, then regulatory action (i.e., prohibition) becomes virtually automatic unless a threshold level of allowable risk has been established. Thus, in the early 1980s, for example, Canadian regulators found that because of their failure to specify such a threshold in rules on disposal of radioactive materials, the ashes of Canadians cremated abroad could not legally cross the border without special permission from the nuclear regulatory authority.[98]

Regulators, and theorists of regulation, use various methods to define a threshold of risk so small that it need not be reduced further. One method is reminiscent of the approach adopted by *Chatam Sofer* and some others, described earlier. This quantitative method involves simply choosing some very low probability as a limit for concern. For example, the (U.S.) Environmental Protection Agency had once determined the acceptable level of benzidine in drinking water as that amount that would place those drinking the water at a one-in-a-hundred-million chance of developing cancer.[99] The city of Long Beach, California, similarly passed a building ordinance on earthquake hazards that defined as acceptable a death risk through earthquake of one person per million exposed in the building per year.[100] But such a quantitative approach is, practically by definition, arbitrary. Some analysts choose the benchmark figure of one in a hundred thousand, rather than a million;[101] who is to say which figure is better? (Recall that similarly R 'Azula'i referred to "once in tens of thousands," whereas R Chayes spoke of "once in millions.")

A second approach to setting risk thresholds corresponds to our understanding of the talmudic dictum "Once many have trampled upon it, 'G-d protects fools.'" An example of this approach is given by

R. H. Mole, a British medical scientist who was writing at a time when, for a number of reasons, civil servants in England were being encouraged to move from the southeastern region (which had very low background levels of radiation) to other portions of the country. Noting the fact that people do not, to use the rabbinic phrase, "concern themselves" with the net change in their level of background radiation when considering whether or not to move, Mole argued, "*A fortiori* experiments on volunteers for medical purposes which involve radiation exposure perhaps 50 or 100 times smaller, corresponding to geographical differences in the annual dose from natural background, not the lifetime's dose, should also be regarded as involving a risk which is truly negligible."[102]

I do not mean to claim that the risk analysts' principle of negligible risk and the rabbinic principle of "trampling" are identical. The risk analyst deals with risks faced by a population, in which even one-in-a-million chances reflect not mere possibilities but eventual casualty figures; his or her judgment must reflect that fact. The rabbinic principle, which we will explore further shortly, applies to risks faced by an individual and judged by that same individual. I think it plausible, therefore, that the rabbinic principle permits much higher risks than any figure that would be felt to be acceptable for a population.

Nonetheless, the parallels are remarkable. It is worthwhile to again return to first principles in considering how they arise. The regime of rights permits persons, under the legal doctrine of "assumption of risk," to voluntarily consent to very great danger. That justification, however, does not cover risks that are, in effect, imposed upon a population, for example, risks that are determined by the design of public policy on issues such as environmental regulation, occupational health, and consumer product safety. In these cases, risks threaten personal safety without being excused by personal consent. Such a regime is driven to find some (low) threshold of permissible risk, so that the activities of life will go on without being paralyzed by ever-growing awareness of risks.

The regime of duties is driven to find a low threshold of permissible risk for much the same reason, although now this threshold applies to individuals—who may not, as reasonable caretakers of their bodies, lawfully consent to personal risks—rather than to populations. Without establishing a level at which risk is low enough that it may be ignored for practical purposes, the activities of life would grind to a halt; as R Basil Herring puts it,

> To insist that a person assiduously avoid every possible situation that might bring him harm would effectively prevent much of normal daily living. Crossing the street could result in one's being run over; eating fish could lead to choking on a bone; and walking alone could result in one's being attacked and injured. How then is one to differentiate between permitted and forbidden "risks"? The answer of the Talmud is that it depends on the accepted conventions of society. Activities that most people engage in with relative ease can be considered permissible, even though there might be some statistical risk involved.[103]

Subjective Aspects of Risk: Definition and Presentation

The Patient's Role in Defining Dangerous Illness

The last major rabbinic topic to be considered relates to a traditional recognition of the subjectivity of risk. The patient's own reactions to risks of suffering, *tza'ar,* and even of danger, *sakana,* are often considered to be legally definitive of those risks that may and may not be undergone by that patient.

With the exception of three laws (murder, idolatry, and extreme sexual misconduct such as incest), the need to protect life supersedes other requirements of the Torah.[104] In particular, even such serious ritual prohibitions as violations of the Sabbath are permitted on behalf of the care and comfort of patients who are dangerously ill.[105] However: Who determines whether a patient is dangerously ill, and what that patient needs? I will quote two such discussions instancing the rabbinic acceptance of the subjectivity of risk. The first deals with the ritual prohibition of eating on Yom Kippur:

Mishna: A sick person is fed [on Yom Kippur] at the bidding of experts; and if there are no experts present, he is fed at his own bidding, until he says: It is enough. [Rashi, s.v. "experts": Should two physicians say that he will be endangered unless he eats.][106]

Gemara: "A sick person is fed at the bidding of experts":

R Yannai said: If a sick person said he needs this, and a doctor says he does not need this, we listen to the sick person. For what reason? "The heart knows the bitterness of its own soul."[107]

—This is obvious! [I.e., why bother saying something so elementary?]

——I would have said [if I had not learned R Yannai's view], "A doctor's view is more authoritative"; this is why he taught that.

If a doctor says he needs this, and the patient says he does not need this, we listen to the doctor. For what reason? He [the patient] is speaking foolishness [tunva]. [Rashi, s.v. tunva: Madness (shtut) on account of his sickness.][108]

The verse that begins "The heart knows the bitterness of its own soul" concludes "and a stranger will not mix within its joy." The Talmud quite frequently quotes fragments of verses, even when the fragment left unquoted is crucial to understanding the interpretation the Talmud assigns to the verse. This is, I think, one of those cases. Taken as a whole, the verse is both asserting a patient's access to his own suffering ("The heart knows") and the inability of outsiders to understand the patient's experience ("and a stranger will not . . . "). Thus its appropriateness as a resolution of the issue under discussion: The patient's view of his own need is accepted ("The heart knows") and that of the doctor is rejected ("and a stranger will not . . . ").

Several separate points on the subjectivity of risk are established in this discussion:

1. The patient is competent to judge the seriousness of his own condition, that is, whether or not it endangers him. (He is

only permitted to eat on this fast day if he is endangered by his illness.)

2. The patient is competent to judge whether his condition requires him to eat.

3. The patient's view that he needs to eat is accepted despite contrary expert objection.

    However, the reliability of the patient's subjective reaction requires that the patient be competent:

4. The doctor's view that the patient needs to eat supersedes the patient's statement that he need not eat, because in this situation we suspect the patient may have been rendered incompetent (i.e., a *shote*) because of his illness.

The second excerpt is concerned with a request by a woman in childbirth during the Sabbath that a lamp be lighted. Such an act violates the ritual prohibition of kindling a fire on the Sabbath, but a woman in childbirth is always considered to be in danger:

> It has been said: If she needed a lamp, her friend lights it for her.
> —But this is obvious! [Rashi: Since preservation of life supersedes the Sabbath.]
> ——This [ruling] is only needed on behalf of a blind woman. We would have said: "Since she cannot see, it is prohibited"; and this teaches us instead, Her mind will be eased by this [ituvei mitva da'ata], by her reasoning: "If I need something, my friend will see that and do it for me" [and it is therefore permitted].[109]

The literary form shared by the two passages reinforces their shared message that the patient's subjective reactions count. In each case, the passage commences with a statement of a ritual violation that is permitted on behalf of an ill person. The statement is then challenged as being obvious, in light of the overwhelming importance Judaism attaches to the protection and preservation of life. In response, the Talmud broadens the meaning of the original, permissive statement, so that it will cover circumstances in which seemingly objective reasons for disregarding the patient's request are superseded by the fact of the request.

"The Heart Knows Its Soul's Bitterness": Scope and Meaning

In the substantial rabbinic literature that discusses these passages and related matters, one preoccupation has been the empirical basis and scope of the statement "The heart knows its soul's bitterness." Is the claim always true? It appears, on its face, to be a "physicalist" principle, and it raises the accompanying problems of reliance upon rabbinic claims of medical fact rather than law and ethics.

The phrase was introduced when discussing a person who wishes to eat on Yom Kippur, and so one late view attempts to limit the principle's scope to that case. A person does not, that is, have any privileged access to knowledge of his body's infirmities, but a person certainly does know how much he hungers.[110] On this understanding, the patient's subjective reaction is ritually controlling for only one "illness," hunger, and only one cure, "food"; not for other illnesses and medical treatments.

This late proposal was in fact considered and rejected by an earlier writer,[111] who was asked whether the Sabbath may be violated to prepare medicine in a case where a patient says he needs it, while a doctor denies that it is needed. Radvaz writes,

> In all cases of illness [and not simply in respect to hunger], we maintain that "the heart knows its soul's bitterness"; for, even though most patients are not expert regarding their own sickness, a minority are expert; lest this patient be one who is expert, we rule leniently on behalf of preservation of life, for we do not rely upon a majority [i.e., a probability greater than 50%] in matters of the preservation of life.

A patient, that is, does not necessarily have superior insight into his condition. But, on the other hand, he may, and legally, that possibility creates a doubt that must be resolved in favor of life. Radvaz here rejects the strong physicalist claim—that patients always know what is best for them—in favor of a weak physicalist claim: They may know what is best. Even that claim, however, may presume too much. Is it always true that patients may know what is best? A further attenuation is offered by R Yisra'el Me'ir Hakohen:

> The Radvaz had written that if an ill person said "I need such-and-such medication" and the doctor said he does not need it, we obey the patient, as we see regarding the fast day of Yom Kippur. In my humble opinion, this is only so when he says that I feel a weakness in such-and-such a part of the body; in that case, they should give him such-and-such a medicine that helps those ill in that part of the body. Then, we certainly listen to him, for "the heart knows its soul's bitterness," is certainly relevant. And even if a doctor should say he does not need any medicine, we do not listen to him. However, if the sickness is known, and the patient says that this medicine will help this sickness, and the doctor says it does not help, it is illogical to listen to the patient and to violate the Sabbath for no reason.[112]

When the principle is understood in this qualified manner, I think problems of "physicalism" have largely dissipated. The principle "The heart knows its own soul's bitterness" is limited to the claim that a patient knows his own *symptoms* (rather than illness) better than anyone else. The inferences drawn above from the Talmud would be modified as follows:

1. The patient is competent to judge the seriousness of his own symptoms.
2. The patient is competent to judge whether his symptoms respond to a given treatment.
3. The patient's view of what provides him with symptomatic relief is accepted over expert objection.

Whether the claims expressed in 1 and 2 are not in fact logical rather than empirical in nature becomes, I think, a difficult question for the philosophy of medicine. Can something be truly said to be a symptom (rather than, e.g., a "sign or marker of illness") if it does not trouble the patient?

If taken as empirical claims, they are at any rate unobjectionable statements of common sense. In combination, the three statements seem to correspond with current medical thinking about the paradigmatic symptom, namely, pain: "If there are discrepancies between a child's report of pain and the observation of a parent or physician, it is best to defer to the child's perspective."[113]

Finally, the empirical import of the principle is limited in one further way. "The heart knows its own soul's bitterness," the patient's privileged access to his own symptoms and symptomatic relief, is a strong enough source of knowledge to overcome ritual requirements. It is not, however, strong enough to overcome directly conflicting expert opinion, as Radvaz concludes in the earlier-quoted responsum:

> I do nonetheless admit that if the wise doctor says that the requested medicine will harm him, we listen to the doctor, even on a non-Sabbath. Insofar as the reason given is that of danger, where have we seen that we rely upon the patient?!—to the contrary, rely upon the doctor!—for he is more expert, and a greater danger will be created if we give the requested medication.[114]

Radvaz may be understood here as alluding to the distinction we have drawn. In many cases, the authority of the patient as reasonable caretaker covers pain, *tza'ar*, but not danger, *sakana*.

The Patient's Fears and Beliefs Create Risk: Another Grounding of Subjectivity

A second line of reasoning regarding the subjectivity of risk has also developed in rabbinic sources, although the fact that it is a distinct principle has not always been recognized (as, for example, in the just-quoted responsum of Radvaz). In addition to accepting that the patient's reaction to symptoms is controlling, many sources consider that the patient's own beliefs and fears are themselves a source of risk, and even danger, of the first order of importance.

This reflects the most natural understanding of the second talmudic passage quoted earlier. There was no objective need for the lamp to be lit; had there been, the midwife attending the woman would have done so without being asked. Nor is the lamp lit because we assume the woman in labor feels that she herself is in need of it—she is blind. It is simply lit, at her request, in order to ease or calm her mind.

The power of this consideration in the literature is affected by a number of variables.[115] One such is the apparent sincerity of the patient's request. A somewhat offbeat example concerned a man who had vowed never again to gamble for money. Subsequent to this, it was claimed, he had begun to suffer from mental illness. He now alleges that his condition is relieved by gambling: Is he permitted to renege on his oath "to relieve his mind"?[116]

We need to consider, too, whether the patient belongs to a class considered to be psychologically "at risk." *Tosfot* state that a woman in childbirth is more prone to become endangered by reason of fear than are other patients, even those suffering from dangerous conditions;[117] that is why the law is particularly lenient in their regard. Another psychologically vulnerable class is made up of those who have taken to their deathbed *[sh'khiv mera']*, who live with the awareness that they will shortly die. The rabbis placed great emphasis upon adhering to the expressed wishes of one who is on his deathbed, altering the law and permitting violations of the usual Sabbath rules so that such a person will be secure in knowing that his final wishes and bequests are being respected.[118] A third class consists of those suffering from mental illness.[119] These variables and classifications are themselves, however, only rough guidelines; it is better to depend upon the judgment of the physicians of the patient, considering matters on a case-by-case basis.[120]

There have been some suggestions made that the weight to be attached to the patient's expression depends upon its reasonableness. Radvaz, for example, explains (on Rambam's behalf) why a man bit by a rabid dog may not eat a lobe of its (of course, nonkosher) liver as a cure (apparently the same homeopathic approach responsible for our phrase "hair of the dog that bit you"). Granted, it is said, this cure is magical and has no scientific validity; still and all, if a patient demands it, perhaps it should be given "to relieve his mind." The answer: "And were this to be permitted to calm the mind [*mishum yituv da'atei*] of the one who was bitten, then take it either way: If he does not know that he is eating the flesh of a dog, his mind would not be relieved; and if he did [know], his soul would despise this, and his illness would continue!"[121] Another such: R Moshe Feinstein rejects the idea that a woman traveling to the hospital to give birth in violation of the Sabbath may be accompanied by her husband or mother "to ease her mind," since there is no reasonable basis for this demand.[122]

I believe, though, that "reasonableness" is only relevant, if at all, to judging permissions under the first principle, "the heart knows its soul's bitterness." It is the very essence of the second principle, "to relieve the mind," that it is the depth of feeling rather than its reasonableness that is in question, and those two qualities are commonly in inverse proportion. Indeed, we have learned from R Feinstein himself that patients who dread treatment, however necessary—even if they dread such elementary matters as nutrition (artificial feeding)—must have those deep feelings respected despite their irrationality:

> It must be given in a manner such that he will not be afraid of it, for if he is afraid of it, *even if this is a matter of sh'tut* [emphasis added], we should not do so, for fear can harm and even kill him, and it would be like killing him with your own hands.[123]

Subjectivity in Practice: An Illustrative Case

However conceptually distinct, in practice the two permissive principles I have described are commonly both present. The authorities are agreed that when the doctors say they have no effective treatment for a patient, yet a patient still demands that he be treated, he should have his demand satisfied (provided that this treatment does not itself represent a serious danger).[124] In such a case, the patient's peace of mind demands the attempt be made; and the sensitive physician continues to hope that he may be wrong after all, and the patient right.

Ethics Consultation: I Shall Please

A Friday afternoon phone call from Dr. E asked for advice concerning a new and difficult problem he faced. A sixty-year-old woman had been left, some years back, with unremitting facial pain after a bout with shingles. She was followed for a long time at the pain clinic of another city hospital, without success. Apparently many means of pain control were attempted, including the ultimate drastic step of severing the trigeminal nerve. Nothing having helped, the woman has felt suicidal, and has in fact attempted suicide twice.

She has now switched hospitals and was referred to a neurologist here. She came with news of a new treatment developed by a Swiss physician, involving intravenous gamma globulin. The neurologist passed her along to Dr. E, an infectious-disease specialist.

Dr. E has assiduously scoured the medical databases and literature, looking for prior experience with this treatment for this condition, without success. He has corresponded with the mysterious Swiss physician and has spoken with him by phone. Dr. E sees no rationale for this treatment, despite the recommendation of the Swiss doctor, who seemed to him to be citing irrelevant comparisons and experience. In addition, IV gamma globulin has real although limited toxicity, described as being about of the order of antibiotics. At the possible (but very unlikely) extreme, it can cause an anaphylactic reaction resulting in death.

He told this to the husband of this patient, who begged Dr. E to do something, to at least give her a placebo (saline water by injection or IV, presumably). (The same suggestion had been made independently by the chief of infectious diseases in conversation with Dr. E.) Dr. E spoke with the hospital's director of professional services, who supported Dr. E's tentative decision not to go along with the patient's unsubstantiated desire for this form of treatment. He had then called me; I asked for some time to think about this, and agreed to get back to him Monday.

I spent part of the weekend talking about this case with two colleagues. There were a lot of questions and uncertainties they mentioned that I could not resolve, having to do with the sequence of events, who was the patient's primary care physician, what treatments had been tried without success and for how long, among many others. Some of the things we didn't know could be quite important and could vitiate any conclusion reached in ignorance of them.

The literature on placebos and their clinical use is of little help in reaching a conclusion, although valuable in clarifying the kinds of considerations to judge and consequences to fear. What happens if a placebo works, for example?—how long should the deception be maintained, can it be successfully maintained, won't the woman feel betrayed and/or humiliated when the truth comes out, and so on? The literature on philosophy and placebos is similarly helpful on background, particularly in pointing out the near identity between the placebo effect and trust in a doctor, but not in reaching a conclusion in this case.

It has always been my feeling that the philosophical and ethical literature on clinical placebos is substantially culture-bound, in ways not recognized; in particular, Sissela Bok's important work, *Lying*,[125] is an expression of the dour Northern European Protestant approach to lying. As a Jew, it seemed to me my culture and religion alike have a less obsessive, and substantially more permissive, stance toward "white lies." Rambam, in laws of theft and loss,[126] lists a number of minor lies that a scrupulously honest person is permitted to commit to save himself and others needless work or embarrassment. In the classic passage of TB *N'darim* 22, we are taught that a person is permitted (or, according to the second view recorded there, required) to "change" what he says—to fib—in order to preserve harmonious family and social relations.[127] It must be admitted that while these place truth-telling in a different light than Bok, they don't really help to resolve this case's perplexities.

Building from a suggestion raised by one colleague, we agreed that the following approach is plausible: After clearly in-

forming the patient of the potential for toxicity, begin treatment with the IV gamma globulin. (This colleague has been
impressed with the fact that IV gamma globulin has worked for
several indications for reasons that remain quite mysterious.) If
she has no relief, that would be the end of the story. If she is relieved to some significant degree, then treat the patient as an N
of 1 in a trial, fiddling with the dose and at times substituting
saline to see whether she responds as well to lower doses or to
pure saline as to the IV gamma globulin. All this can and needs
to be explained to her beforehand, and done with her consent:
Since the treatment has toxicity, since there is very little experience with this treatment for this condition, since we do not
know how she as an individual will respond, she will be treated
on different doses and at times will be given saline. She will be
consenting to not being informed of when the dosage is changing, because her knowledge would make it impossible for us to
discover what the lowest possible effective dose of treatment will
be for her. In this way, the issue has become one of consented
nondisclosure rather than deception. Alternatively, all agreed
that if the physician was uncomfortable with this maneuver, he
could simply decline to satisfy the patient's desire. Speaking
with Dr. D on Monday, he agreed to try the stratagem. He will
be away for a couple of days and will try to begin this approach
on Thursday.

Conclusion: Summarizing *Halakhic* Principles of Personal Medical Decision Making

In the discussion of consent, the idea of responsibility for the self was
introduced. There I argued that while the patient does not "own" his
own body, he is in fact in the legal position of guardianship over his
own body. As such, he is required to care for his body, through taking
thought over medical choices as well as through his deeds. He needs
to act with prudence, avoiding negligence *[p'shi'a]*; that is, he needs to
act as a reasonable caretaker would act.

That verbal formula is useful as a conceptual construct and, perhaps, when judging conduct in the abstract, or in judging another's conduct. It is not, however, of much practical use from the first-party perspective, from my own point of view when I am faced with a particular choice. How am I, as a reasonable caretaker, supposed to reason about this choice? The approach that emerges from the material presented here yields no simple formula, but rather a number of guidelines and considerations that I am obliged to consider. The following principles are among them.

The General Principle: The Requirement to Safeguard Life and Health. Overall, I am required as a responsible caretaker to avoid all forms of risk: serious risk of death, *sakana,* and risks that involve pain, suffering, and wounding, *tza'ar.*

Principles Regarding Tza'ar

- *Tza'ar's* subjectivity: My own perception of *tza'ar,* of the impact that illness has upon my life (through direct physical pain or more broadly), supersedes the judgment of others, including my physician or other experts.
- Minimizing *tza'ar:* I am permitted, and perhaps obliged, to consider the overall impact my decision will have upon my life with respect to *tza'ar,* and to act rationally in minimizing *tza'ar,* by (for example) undergoing some pain in the short run to prevent greater suffering in the long run.
- Minimizing factors that cause *tza'ar:* In performing such an analysis, I am permitted, and perhaps required, to consider not simply *tza'ar* itself but other factors that shall have an impact on *tza'ar,* including the personal financial implications of my decision.

Principles Regarding Sakana

- Minimizing *sakana:* I am required to be risk-averse with regard to *sakana,* serious danger to life, and to recognize that expert estimations of *sakana* are more reliable than my own estimation. This does not, however, imply that my task as a reasonable caretaker is fulfilled by automatic avoidance of all such risk.

- Threshold of *sakana:* The minor risks associated with the ordinary activities of life may be ignored. Risks to life that are highly improbable and, as such, are ignored on an everyday basis by prudent people do not come within the class of *sakana* that must be avoided.
- *Sakana* and social functioning: I may subject myself to a substantially higher level of risk than that faced by most persons in ordinary life if I need to do so to secure my ability to function socially, for example, through my livelihood.
- *Sakana* and personal choices:
  1. I should judge my choices realistically, considering my own individuality and especially psychological vulnerability. Under conditions of extreme pressure, I should be aware that these psychological propensities, if ignored, may place me at greater risk than other objective features of the situation.
  2. While I am always permitted, and perhaps obliged, to attempt through my choices to reduce the *tza'ar* that I experience and the *sakana* that I face, such decisions are personal ones and may be made in ways that express the values that I hold and my general approach to life.
  3. The leeway that I have to express my values and lifestyle in these choices becomes most broad and important when making decisions while facing death, either because death is imminent or because I suffer from a disease that is expected to kill me within the year.

Implicit within each of these principles is the need any reasonable caretaker has to exercise intelligence and curiosity in clarifying the nature and consequences of the choices that he or she faces. This includes, of course, the sort of information that we are accustomed to include under the rubric of "informed consent." The requirement, however, goes well beyond that. When understood as a right, informed consent speaks to the conscientious physician's supplying information to the patient. In Judaism's regime of duty, the reasonable caretaker is obliged to assimilate that information and to relate it to his or her own personal values and life-plans. The reasonable caretaker is thus subject to the philosopher's injunction: Know thyself.

Endnotes

1. *Gesher Hachayim* 1, chapter 1, section 2.2.
2. TB *Yoma* 83a.
3. TB *Yoma* 84b.
4. Responsa *Sh'vut Ya'akov* 3, no. 75.
5. Rambam, *Hilkhot Rotzei'ach* 2.7.
6. On *Orach Chaim,* section 229.
7. Responsa *Tzitz Eli'ezer* 4, section 13; compare with R Y. Schmelkes, Responsa *Beit Yitzchak, Yore Dei'a* 2, section 162, part 3.*
8. 2 Kings 7.4.
9. TB *Avoda Zara* 27b.
10. See R Moshe Feinstein, Responsa *Igrot Moshe, Choshen Mishpat* 2, section 68.
11. In fact, the prohibition upon using the services of an idolater is limited to cases of dangerous illness.*
12. Joseph Shatzmiller, *Jews, Medicine, and Medieval Society* (Berkeley: University of California Press, 1994): 92–93.*
13. TB *Shabbat* 33b.*
14. R Moshe Feinstein, Responsa *Igrot Moshe, Yore Dei'a* 2, section 174.
15. See R Moshe Feinstein, *Igrot Moshe, Choshen Mishpat* 2, section 73; see also R Eli'ezer Waldenberg, Responsa *Tzitz Eli'ezer,* vol. 10, section 25.*
16. *Tzitz Eli'ezer,* vol. 10, section 25.*
17. Responsa *Igrot Moshe, Choshen Mishpat* 2, section 73.
18. Responsa *Tzitz Eli'ezer,* vol. 10, section 25; compare R Chayim Ozer Gorodzinsky, Responsa *Achi'ezer,* vol. 2, part 16, no. 6. See also R Leivi Yitzchak Halperin, "Regarding an Operation: Is it Permissible to Accept Danger for the Sake of Relief . . . " [in Hebrew] in *Sefer Halakha Ur'fu'a* 3, ed. R Moshe Hershler (Jerusalem: Regensberg Institute, 1983): 140–141.*
19. TB *Sanhedrin* 90.
20. R Moshe Feinstein in *Halakha Ur'fu'a* (Sefer Regensburg), vol. 1, op. cit., "Endangering Temporary Life on Behalf of Possible Lengthening

Life," 131–142, at 135, 136, 137; also in *Igrot Moshe, Choshen Mishpat* 2, section 73.

21. R Shlomo Zalman Auerbach, quoted and discussed in Abraham S. Abraham, *Nishmat Avraham, Yore Dei'a* 155, 47–48.

22. Compare R Moshe Feinstein, *Igrot Moshe, Choshen Mishpat* 2, section 73; compare also R Shlomo Zalman Auerbach, quoted in *Nishmat Avraham, Yore Dei'a* 155, 47, note 29.*

23. R Leivi Yitzchak Halperin (1983): 140–141.*

24. Ramban, *Torat Ha'adam*, in *Kitvei Rabenu Moshe ben Nachman*, vol. 2, ed. R Chaim Dov Chavel (Tel Aviv: Mossad Harav Kood, 1963): 40–41.

25. Lev. 19.18.

26. Lev. 24.21.

27. TB *Sanhedrin* 84b.

28. See *Shulchan Arukh, Yore Dei'a* 241.3, and Rambam, *Hilkhot Mamrim* 5.7, and commentators there.

29. This is taken by some writers as an indication that Ramban derives the commandment to heal from this verse, rather than from the commandment to return lost property, as did Rambam; see "The Duty to Heal" in Section 2.*

30. Ramban, *Torat Ha'adam*, pp. 41 ff.; emphases added. This view is followed and elaborated by Ran *(Chidushei HaRan,* TB *Sanhedrin* 84b, s.v. *Rav lo shavak librei).**

31. See Benjamin Freedman, "Cohort-Specific Consent: An Honest Approach to Phase I Clinical Cancer Studies," *IRB: A Review of Human Subjects Research* 12, no. 1 (1990): 5–7.*

32. TB *Sota* 20a.

33. TB *B'rakhot* 5b.

34. TB *K'tubot* 104a.

35. Ran on TB *N'darim* 40b.

36. Compare with R Leivi Yitzchak Halperin (1983): 142.*

37. *Orach Chaim* 328.

38. TB *K'tubot* 62a.

39. R Eli'ezer Waldenberg, Responsa *Tzitz Eli'ezer* 13, section 87; compare too *Tzitz Eli'ezer* 12, section 18 (7).*

40. R Moshe Feinstein, Responsa *Igrot Moshe, Choshen Mishpat* 2, sec-

tion 73, part 9; see later on the possibility that R Feinstein did not view the risk common to all operations as morally considerable.

41. R Moshe Feinstein, Responsa *Igrot Moshe, Choshen Mishpat* 2, section 73; emphasis added.

42. See note 33. Compare also *Nishmat Avraham, Yore Dei'a* 155, pp. 48–49.*

43. R Shlomo Zalman Auerbach in *Minchat Shlomo*, section 91, part 24.

44. R Moshe Feinstein, Responsa *Igrot Moshe, Choshen Mishpat* 2, section 74.

45. The story, recounted in several Midrashic sources, is most familiar through compilations of these sources included in the liturgy, e.g., the *Ele ezk'ra* portion of Yom Kippur's *Musaf* prayer.

46. TB *Bava Kamma* 91b.

47. Gen. 9.5.

48. Note *Tosfot*, TB *Bava Kamma* 91b, s.v. *Ela hai tana.**

49. Num. 6.11.

50. TY *Kidushin* 4.12.

51. Another example of a legal distinction between harm and danger occurs in respect of filial obligation; see *Sefer Chasidim*, section 234.*

52. *Nishmat Avraham, Yore Dei'a* 155, p. 49.

53. Responsa *Chelkat Ya'akov* 3, section 11; R Moshe Feinstein, *Halakha Ur'fu'a*, vol. 1, p. 323; *Sh'arim M'tzuyanim B'halakha*, section 190; R Jakobovitz, *Noam*, vol. 6, p. 273.

54. R Eli'ezer Waldenberg, Responsa *Tzitz Eli'ezer* 11, section 41; Responsa *Minchat Yitzchak* 6, section 105.

55. In his note 45.

56. *Hilkhot Chovel Umazik* 5:1.

57. Responsa *Minchat Yitzchak* 6, section 105, part 2.

58. R Moshe Feinstein, "An Operation upon a Girl for Her Self-Beautification," in *Halakha Ur'fu'a*, vol. 1, ed. R Moshe Hershler (Jerusalem: Regensberg Institute, 1980): 323–327.

59. TB *Shabbat* 50b, s.v. *Bishvil.*

60. R Eli'ezer Waldenberg, Responsa *Tzitz Eli'ezer* 11, section 41.

61. See R Moshe Feinstein in *Halakha Ur'fu'a*, vol. 1, "Endangering Temporary Life on Behalf of Possible Lengthening Life," 131–142, at 137–138.*

62. Responsa *Binyan Tziyon,* section 137.

63. On the question of whether the blessing may be recited by a person who had negligently become ill, see Responsa *Yechave Da'at* 4, section 14.

64. Ibid.*

65. Deut. 24.15.

66. TB *Bava Metzi'a* 112a.

67. Responsa *Noda BiYehuda, Yore Dei'a Tenina,* section 10; and compare *Sefer Chasidim,* section 341.*

68. See R Tzvi Beer, *Imrei Tzvi* on TB *Bava Kamma* 91b.*

69. R Moshe Feinstein, Responsa *Igrot Moshe, Choshen Mishpat* 1, section 104.

70. See R Jakobovits's reasoning in Prof. Abraham's *Nishmat Avraham, Yore Dei'a* 155; see also *Sefer Chasidim,* section 341.*

71. Compare with Benjamin Freedman, *Consensuality, Regulation and Societal Risk* (Report contracted by the Law Reform Commission of Canada, Project on Protection of Life, Health, and the Environment, 1984).

72. Compare with Benjamin Freedman, "Health Care Workers' Occupational Exposure to HIV: Obligations to Care and Entitlements from Care," in *Perspectives on AIDS: Ethical and Social Issues,* ed. Christine Overall with William P. Zion (New York: Oxford University Press, 1991): 91–105.

73. *Reibl v. Hughes,* Supreme Court of Canada, 114 DLR 3d 1-35, Oct. 7, 1980, per Laskin CJ.

74. R Moshe Feinstein (1980): 323–327.

75. Responsa *Chatam Sofer* 2, *Yore Dei'a,* section 338.*

76. Responsa *Maharatz Chayot,* section 52.

77. Responsa *Chayim Sha'al* 2, section 25.

78. Compare: Responsa *Chayim Sha'al* 2, section 25, part 2; and R Moshe Feinstein, Responsa *Igrot Moshe, Yore Dei'a* 2, section 174.*

79. TB *Shabbat* 129b.

80. Friday having a *zugot* hour, the eighteenth, in the daytime, and the day being "governed" by Mars, *Ma'adim.*

81. Ps. 116.6.

82. See TB *Nida* 31a; TB *K'tubot* 21b; TB *'Azoda Zara* 30b.*

83. Rava's view in TB *P'sachim* 64b. See Responsa *Rashba* 1, section 403 for a legal application.

84. Responsa *Yehuda Ya'ale,* vol. 1, *Yore Dei'a* 222, s.v. *v'khol zeh leR Mei'ir.**

85. Compare Responsa *Shivat Tziyon,* section 54, s.v. *v'hinei ra'iti.**

86. Responsa *Ya'avetz* 1, section 14, s.v. *ve'im tomar.**

87. R Eli'ezer Waldenberg's view in Responsa *Tzitz Eli'ezer,* vol. 9, section 17, *Kuntres R'fua B'Shabbat,* chapter 2.*

88. See Responsa *Yosef Ometz,* section 37; Responsa *Chatam Sofer* 1, *Orach Chayim,* section 23; Responsa *'Ezrat Kohen, Even Ha'ezer,* section 6.*

89. Compare with R Moshe Feinstein, Responsa *Igrot Moshe, Yore Dei'a* 3, section 36; also, R Eliezer Waldenberg, Responsa *Tzitz Eli'ezer* 10, section 25, s.v. *"perek";* and Responsa R Eliyahu Mizrachi section 22; Rulings of the (Israeli) Rabbinic Courts, 7, p. 156, s.v. *yesod v'asmakhta.**

90. R Eli'ezer Waldenberg, Responsa *Tzitz Eli'ezer* 15, section 37, s.v. *Bi'ytera.*

91. Ibid.*

92. Compare *Nishmat Avraham, Yore Dei'a* 155, pp. 48–49.*

93. Basil Herring, *Jewish Ethics and Halakha for Our Time,* vol. 1 (New York: Ktav , 1984): 230.

94. See Marcus Jastrow, *A Dictionary of the Targumim* (reprinted in Israel by Hillel Press, no date), s.v. *Dush; mitzvot* that one is *dosh* by his heel: TB *Avoda Zara* 18a.

95. TB *K'tubot* 62a.

96. See my *Consensuality, Regulation and Societal Risk* (Report contracted by the Law Reform Commission of Canada Project on Protection of Life, Health, and the Environment, 1984): 68 ff.; "Philosophical Considerations Concerning Types and Thresholds of Risk," in *Environmental Health Risks: Assessment and Management,* ed. R. Stephen MacColl (Waterloo: University of Waterloo Press, 1987): 305–317; "Starr Gazing: Philosophical and Political Issues Raised by Historically Revealed Preference Theories of Acceptable Risk," in *Total Risk and Benefit Impact of Energy Alternatives,* ed. H. D. Sharma (Waterloo: University of Waterloo Press, 1990): 97; William W. Lowrance, *Of Acceptable Risk* (Los Altos, CA: William Kaufman Inc., 1976): 21.

98. "Easing of Rules for Radiation Disposal Studied," *Toronto Globe and Mail,* Nov. 4 (1981): A4.

99. See Lowrance (1976): 135–136.

100. John H. Wiggins Jr., "Earthquake Safety in the City of Long Beach Based on the Concept of Balanced Risk," in *Perspectives on Benefit-Risk Decision Making* (Washington, D.C.: National Academy of Engineering, 1972): 88.

101. See Freedman (1984): "Risk," note 76.*

102. R. H. Mole, "Accepting Risks for Other People," *Proceedings of the Royal Society of Medicine* 69 (1976): 108.

103. Herring (1984): 230.

104. TB *Sanhedrin* 74a.

105. TB *Yoma* 85b.

106. TB *Yoma* 82a.

107. Pro. 14.10.

108. TB *Yoma* 83a.*

109. TB *Shabbat* 128b.

110. Responsa *S'ridei Eish* 2, section 158.

111. Responsa *Radvaz*, vol. 4, section 66.

112. R Yisrael Meir Hakohen (better known eponymously as "the Chafetz Chaim") in *Mishne Berura, Orach Chayim,* section 328, paragraph 10, in *Be'ur Halakha,* s.v. *V'rophei echad.*

113. G. A. Walco, R. C. Cassidy, and N. L. Schechter, "Pain, Hurt, and Harm—The Ethics of Pain Control in Infants and Children," *New England Journal of Medicine* 331 (1994): 541–544.

114. Responsa *Radvaz* 4, section 66.

115. See R Eli'ezer Waldenberg, Responsa *Tzitz Eli'ezer,* monograph *M'shivat Nefesh,* chapter 9 (in his vol. 8, section 15).*

116. See Responsa of Rashba that are attributed to Ramban, section 281.

117. *Tosfot,* TB *Shabbat* 128b, s.v. *Ka mashma lan.*

118. See TB *Bava Batra* 156b.

119. See Responsa of Rashba that are attributed to Ramban, section 281.

120. R Eli'ezer Waldenberg, Responsa *Tzitz Eli'ezer,* monograph *M'shivat Nefesh,* chapter 9 (in his vol 8, section 15).

121. Responsa *Radvaz* 5, section 153, dealing with the violation of Sabbath by carrying such healing talismans as the tooth of a fox or a nail from a crucifixion.

122. R Moshe Feinstein, Responsa *Igrot Moshe, Orach Chayim* 1, section 132.

123. R Moshe Feinstein, Responsa *Igrot Moshe, Choshen Mishpat* 2, section 73, part 5.

124. Responsa *Radbaz,* vol. 4, section 66; R Eli'ezer Waldenberg, in his monograph *Kuntres M'shivat Nefesh,* chapter 8 in his *Tzitz Eli'ezer,* vol. 8, section 15; R Yisrael Meir Hakohen, in *Mishne Berura,* commentary on *Orach Chayim,* section 328, paragraph 10, in *Bei'ur Halakha,* s.v. *V'rophe echad;* R Moshe Feinstein, Responsa *Igrot Moshe, Choshen Mishpat* 2, section 74.

125. Sissela Bok, *Lying: Moral Choice in Public and Private Life* (New York: Pantheon, 1978).

126. Chapter 14.

127. See also TB *Y'vamot* 65b. The view is also found, with some differences, in *Derekh Eretz Zuta, Perek Hashalom.* For discussion and further references see Moshe Halevi Spero, *Handbook of Psychotherapy and Jewish Ethics* (Jerusalem: Feldheim, 1986): 138, note 86.

Next Steps in Healing and Duty

A famous tale: A gentile approached the rabbis, stating that he would convert on condition that he be taught the entire Torah while standing upon one foot. Two reactions are recorded. Shammai beat him with a stick and drove him away. Hillel accepted the challenge and said: "That which is hateful for you, do not do to your fellow. That is the whole of Torah; all the rest, simply commentary. Go and study!"

It would be helpful to be able to present, at the close of this very lengthy discussion, a unified theory of Jewish bioethics, in the form of a simple principle or set of principles. But that task is beyond me. Nor could I simply adapt Hillel's elegant expression. For one thing, Hillel presumed that we know what we want (or at least, find hateful). As was demonstrated in the cases developed in the previous section on risk, we cannot always know that. In health care more than in many other areas of life, choice is often a matter of judging among evils. For another, Hillel could assume that the gentile will seek out proper instruction in how to interpret the maxim. Such resources are scarce nowadays.

If there is no single principle, there is, I think, a unifying theme that is evident in this work—that is, the power of the concept of duty in providing new light upon old issues in bioethics. Beginning with the idea of an ethics consultation, we have seen how the model of duty enables us to reconceptualize the role sought and played by patient or family member, health care provider, and indeed bioethicist as well. A mutual recognition on the part of participants that each is seeking to fulfill the claims of duty provides new insight into who should be involved in an ethics consultation, how it should be accomplished, and what counts as a successful resolution to the presenting problem. Duty recurred in the following sections: in helping to analyze the basis and nature of a family member's participation in health care decisions on behalf of an incompetent relative; in grounding, for Judaism as well as (potentially) other religious traditions of stewardship, the notion of informed consent as a necessary preliminary to treating competent persons; and in delineating the kinds of considerations such a person should explore in determining what forms of medical treatment to accept. The theme of duty also comes into play in describing the social role a concept like competency plays within the Jewish tradition.

This work has taken individual decisions about health care as the fundamental "problem" of bioethics, the basic unit with which bioethics begins: On what basis is a particular decision about medical or nursing care justified? All of the foregoing may be seen as addressed to a preliminary response to that question. The Prologue, on ethics consultation, asked how we are to understand a discussion between persons on that fundamental question. The sections on consent and risk addressed this problem as it is faced by competent persons; on family, as it is seen by those who speak on behalf of incompetent persons. The section on competence attempted to clarify the marks of distinction between those classes of persons.

It is in this sense that I have claimed to provide the foundations for one Jewish approach to bioethics. Establishing a foundation is a first step, however. It is of little use without erecting a structure, and the structure, in turn, must be furnished. What would be the next steps involved in fleshing out this approach to bioethics?

It could be thought that what is needed is a refinement of the work already begun. In particular, I have avoided discussing some difficult puzzle cases, in which some of the principles established work at cross purposes to others: when, for example, a decision to prolong the life of an incompetent person will extend suffering or engender indignity.

Certainly, such work is needed. Without some effort at prioritizing the ethical principles with which we work, our decisions rest upon a shaky foundation. But I think it is a mistake to believe that a complete and final prioritization is possible. Such an achievement would be an ethical Pyrrhic victory. It would, in principle, eliminate the need for the subject matter of ethics itself: human judgment.

Be that as it may, however, it is certainly a mistake to think that refinement of the approach to the basic bioethical question is all that is needed. Health care is provided within a context, and the next steps require that we explore that context. Let me give some examples of what I mean.

In the provision of health care itself, new relationships are formed that require their own ethical analysis. This work has not dealt with such aspects of the doctor-patient relationship as, for example, confidentiality, truth-telling (except insofar as required by informed consent), or negligence. Nor has it dealt, except in the most preliminary way, with the ethics of other relationships: for example, ethicist–health care proxy, or rabbi–health care proxy.

Certain kinds of care raise their own characteristic, and sometimes unique, ethical problems. Technologically assisted reproduction is one example; organ transplantation, whether the donor be living or dead, another. Both examples are useful in pointing out society's web of interconnectedness, the way in which an individual's decision about health care may both express and help to create relationships to others within society. Abortion and the definition of death can be seen that way as well. Among other issues, they raise the question of the boundaries of social membership and human responsibility.

This work has not dealt with "macro" issues at all, those that are raised by health care policy, including the increasingly prominent issues associated with the allocation of health resources. Jewish sources have pertinent points to make about these issues as well, in discussions that directly define the nature of community responsibility to provide health care as well as preventive services. Moreover, other legal concepts need to be brought analogically to bear, for example, the duty and limits of community provisions for charity and welfare.

Finally, Judaism as well as other religious traditions may provide a perspective that is broadly lacking in current bioethical discussion and yet is badly needed. Some of the new issues being faced, associated with ecology, for example, and genetic manipulation, are drained of their most profound significance when understood in terms of individual rights and private transactions. Religion can provide a fuller understanding, by placing the questions raised within a global and even cosmic context. Any Jewish attempt to understand genetic technology, for example, must do so from within an understanding of the Genesis narrative, with its repeated emphasis upon creation's being effected by the establishment of discrete biological species, each of which shall reproduce after its own kind.[1]

These further explorations, however, are not the work of one book, or of one author.

Endnote

1. On this, see Benjamin Freedman, "Leviticus and DNA: A Very Old Look at a Very New Problem," *Journal of Religious Ethics* 8, no. 1 (1980); and Benjamin Freedman and Marie-Claude Goulet, "New Creations?" (case commentary), *Hastings Center Report* 21, no. 1 (1991): 34–35.

Sources of Jewish Law

1. Hebrew Bible (~1500 BCE–~400 BE). Traditional written law divided into three sections: *Torah* (Pentateuch): Genesis, Exodus, Leviticus, Numbers, and Deuteronomy; *Nevi'im* (Prophets): e.g., Joshua, Kings, Isaiah, Jeremiah, and Ezekiel; and *Ketubim* (Writings): e.g., Psalms, Proverbs, Song of Songs, Lamentations, and Ecclesiastes.

2. Talmud (Mishna and Gemara; two collections—one developed in Palestine, one in Babylon). Mishna (200 CE): Traditional written compilation of Oral Law that is divided into six Orders: *Zera'im, Mo'ed, Nashim, Nezikin, Kodshim,* and *Toharot.* Gemara (200 CE–~500 CE): Rabbinic discussions flowing from Mishna that are further divided into roughly sixty tractates: e.g., *Sanhedrin, Avot, Bava Batra, Avoda Zara, Bava, Kamma, Yoma, Brakhot, Baca Metz'ia, Arachin, Shabbat,* and *Gittin.*

3. Rashi: R Shlomo Yitzchaki (1040–1105). The most important and influential talmudic commentator. Also *Tosfot* (additions): a group of scholars who continued Rashi's tradition of talmudic commentary in the twelfth and thirteenth centuries in France and Germany.

4. Rambam, or Maimonides (1135–1204). Summarized the talmudic legal rulings into the great codification, the *Mishne Tora.*

5. The *Shulkhan Aruch.* The culmination of a great period of code-making among European authorities, including the *Tur* of R Yaakov ben Asher, which is the code of R Yosef Karo (1488–1575) split into four major thematic divisions.

6. Responsa (medieval period to present). This vast body of literature has been the main source for detailed rabbinic discussion and innovation in modern times.

Glossary

bein adam l'chaveiro "Between a man and his friend"

bein adam lamakom "Between a man and the Omnipresent"

chavala Wounding

chayav Duty-bound

chayei olam Lasting life, eternal life

chayei sha'a "Fleeting life"

Chida Acronym for eighteenth-century Italian R Chayim Yosef David 'Azula'i

chovah Strict obligation

ch'shash sakana Doubtful risk

get A bill of divorcement

Gemara A compilation of rabbinic discussions all of which originate with questions associated with the interpretation of the Mishna

goses One who is moribund (near death)

halakha A legal ruling; a chapter subdivision in the Talmud Yerushalmi

Halakha The corpus of Jewish law

hishameir "Take care" (of oneself)

ketuba A marriage contract

kibud Respectful service, dutiful service

Mishna A compilation of rabbinic legal rulings whose editing was completed by the year 200 CE

Mishne Tora Codification of Jewish law by Rambam (1135–1204); divided into fourteen books

mitzva Deed performed according to one's obligaton or duty; a good deed

morah Reverent obedience

nichpe Epileptic

nidche Suppressed

nishtatek Speechless

patur Inculpable

peti Mentally handicapped; a "fool"

peti b'yoter Profoundly intellectually disabled

piku'ach nefesh Rescue of a soul; saving a life

p'shia Negligence

Rambam (1135–1204) Acronym for R Moshe ben Maimon (Maimonides); noted physician, halakhist; author of *Mishne Tora* and the *Guide of the Perplexed;* worked mainly in Spain and Egypt

Ramban (1194–1270) Acronym for R Moshe ben Nachman (Nachmanides); Talmudist, Cabbalist, and teacher

Rashi (1040–1105) Acronym for French rabbi R Shlomo Yitzchaki; the most influential commentator on the Talmud

refuah b'duka ug'mura Definitive and proven treatment

responsa Compilations of responses by rabbinic authors from the early medieval period to the present to questions posed of them regarding Jewish law; the main source for detailed rabbinic discussion and innovation

sakana Danger; risk

shomeir Caretaker; pl. *shomrim*

shota A madwoman; a female *shote*

shote One who suffers from mental illness; one who is legally incompetent

shtut Madness

Shulchan Arukh Codification of Jewish law by R Yosef Karo (1488–1575); split into four main thematic divisions

Sh'vut Ya'akov Book of responsa

written by R Ya'ako Reisher (1670–1733)

Talmud The combination of the Mishna and the Gemara

Talmud Bavli (TB) The Babylonian Talmud

Talmud Yerushalmi (TY) The Jerusalem Talmud

Tosfot "Additions"; collection of talmudic commentaries from twelfth-century France and Germany

tza'ar Pain

Tur Classic halakhic text, written by R Ya'akov ben Asher (1275–1340)

Tzitz Eli'ezer Collection of responsa by R Eli'ezer Waldenberg

Zohar The "book of Splendour"— central text of medieval mysticism (Cabbalah), thirteenth century

Index